Contents

Introduction

Welcome to the Health and Social Care Level 3 Dementia Care handbook!

Older people, particularly those over 80 years, are the fastest growing age group in the UK population. This group also has the highest risk of developing dementia-based conditions. You can develop dementia at any age, though the risk increases as you get older. About 20 per cent of people over the age of 80 years develop one form of dementia or another. This handbook isn't about dementia as an illness or a condition, though. It is about ways of caring for and supporting people living with dementia.

In the early stages of a dementia-based condition, some people can manage without outside help and are able to continue living at home. As the condition progresses, virtually all individuals with dementia require some level of care and support to cope with daily living. Individuals with dementia need to be cared for and supported by people who understand what is happening to them.

Health and social care workers who practice in dementia care settings or who provide dementia care and support in the community need to be able to use an empathetic, person-centred approach that focuses on the quality of life, dignity and personhood of individuals with dementia. This handbook emphasises the importance of treating every individual with dementia as a unique, valued adult in their own right, regardless of the way dementia affects them. It explains what a person-centred approach involves and what you need to do to demonstrate that you have the skills to work in a person-centred way.

How is the book organised?

The book consists of five chapters and a resources section.

▶ Each chapter of the book covers one or more of the units that make up the Level 3 Award in Awareness of Dementia Care or the Level 3 Certificate in Dementia Care.

▶ Each chapter is divided into different sections, which are matched to the specifications for the Level 3 qualifications. Each section provides you with a focused and manageable chunk of learning.

Overall, the chapters cover all of the learning and assessment requirements of the Level 3 Award and Certificate qualifications.

How is assessment covered?

In order to achieve your Level 3 Award, you will need to provide evidence of your knowledge and understanding of dementia care as well as your practical competence as a dementia care worker in a real work environment. Each chapter of this book ends with a checklist of 'What you need to know' and 'What you need to do' in order to successfully complete the units that a chapter covers. This checklist will help you keep track of your progress.

The suggested assessment tasks in each chapter will help you gather the evidence you need for each unit. Your tutor or assessor will help you to plan your work in order to meet the overall assessment requirements of your target qualification.

We hope that the material in this handbook is accessible, interesting and inspires you to pursue a rewarding career caring for and supporting individuals with dementia. Good luck with your course and your future career!

Mark Walsh, Elaine Millar, John Rowe and Ann Mitchell

Qualification information

The book has been written to cover the:

▶ Level 3 Award in Awareness of Dementia qualification

▶ Level 3 Certificate in Dementia Care qualification

Health and Social Care

Level 3 Dementia Care Award and Certificate

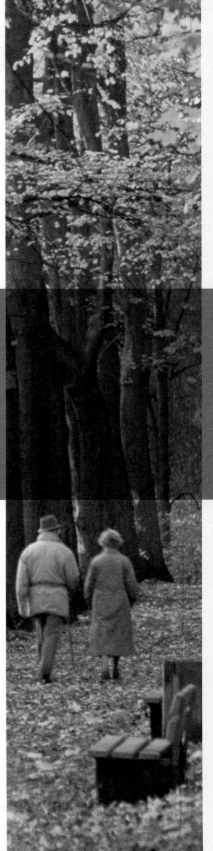

Mark Walsh · Elaine Millar · John Rowe · Ann Mitchell

Published by Collins Education
An imprint of HarperCollins*Publishers*
77–85 Fulham Palace Road
Hammersmith
London
W6 8JB

Browse the complete Collins Education catalogue at
www.collinseducation.com

10 9 8 7 6 5 4 3 2 1

ISBN 978-0-00-746872-0

Mark Walsh, Elaine Millar, John Rowe and Ann Mitchell assert their moral rights
to be identified as the authors of this work.

British Library Cataloguing in Publication Data

A Catalogue record for this publication is available from the British Library.

Project managed by Caroline Low
Edited by Jan Doorly and Matthew Hammond
Index by Annie Dilworth
Picture research by Matthew Hammond
Design and typesetting by Jouve India Private Ltd.
Illustrations by Ann Paganuzzi
Cover design by Angela English
Printed and bound in Italy by Lego

Every effort has been made to contact copyright holders but if any have been
inadvertently overlooked, the publishers will be pleased to make the necessary
arrangements at the first opportunity.

All Crown Copyright Material is produced with permission of the Controller,
Office of Public Sector Information (OPSI)

The units that make up the Level 3 Award provide learners new to dementia care work or those preparing for employment in this area with a solid awareness of dementia care issues. The knowledge gained through the achievement of the Award qualification can also be used to demonstrate competence in the Level 3 Certificate in Dementia Care. This qualification is aimed at those who are already working in care roles with individuals with dementia. It provides learners with an opportunity to have their practical competence as dementia care workers assessed.

Level 3 Award in Awareness of Dementia

Learners aiming to achieve a Level 3 Award in Awareness of Dementia must complete and pass the four mandatory units listed below.

Unit code	Mandatory units	Credits	Book chapter
DEM 301	Understand the process and experience of dementia	3	1
DEM 305	Understand the administration of medication to individuals with dementia using a person-centred approach	2	4
DEM 308	Understand the role of communication and interactions with individuals who have dementia	3	2
DEM 310	Understand the diversity of individuals with dementia and the importance of inclusion	3	3

Level 3 Certificate in Dementia Care

Learners aiming to achieve a Level 3 Certificate in Dementia Care must complete and pass the four mandatory units and the three optional units listed below. (A range of additional optional units can also be taken to achieve the Level 3 Certificate, but are not covered by this handbook.)

Unit code	Mandatory units	Credits	Book chapter
DEM 301	Understand the process and experience of dementia	3	1
DEM 304	Enable rights and choices of individuals with dementia while minimising risks	4	3
DEM 312	Understand and enable interaction and communication with individuals who have with dementia	4	2
DEM 313	Equality, diversity and inclusion in dementia care practice	4	3
Unit code	Optional units	Credits	Book chapter
DEM 302	Understand and meet the nutritional requirements of individuals with dementia	3	5
DEM 305	Understand the administration of medication to individuals with dementia using a person-centred approach	2	4
HSC 3047	Support the use of medication in social care settings	5	4

The achievement of units from both the Award and the Certificate qualifications can be used towards the achievement of the Level 3 Diploma in Health and Social Care (Adults) for England or the Level 3 Diploma in Health and Social Care (Adults) for Wales and Northern Ireland.

1 | The process and experience of dementia

DEM 301
LO1 Understand the neurology of dementia

▶ Describe a range of causes of dementia syndrome

▶ Describe the types of memory impairment commonly experienced by individuals with dementia

▶ Explain the way that individuals process information with reference to the abilities and limitations of individuals with dementia

▶ Explain how other factors can cause changes in an individual's condition that may not be attributable to dementia

▶ Explain why the abilities and needs of an individual with dementia may fluctuate

DEM 301
LO2 Understand the impact of recognition and diagnosis of dementia

▶ Describe the impact of early diagnosis and follow-up to diagnosis

▶ Explain the importance of recording possible signs or symptoms of dementia in an individual in line with agreed ways of working

▶ Explain the process of reporting possible signs of dementia within agreed ways of working

▶ Describe the possible impact of receiving a diagnosis of dementia on the individual, their family and friends

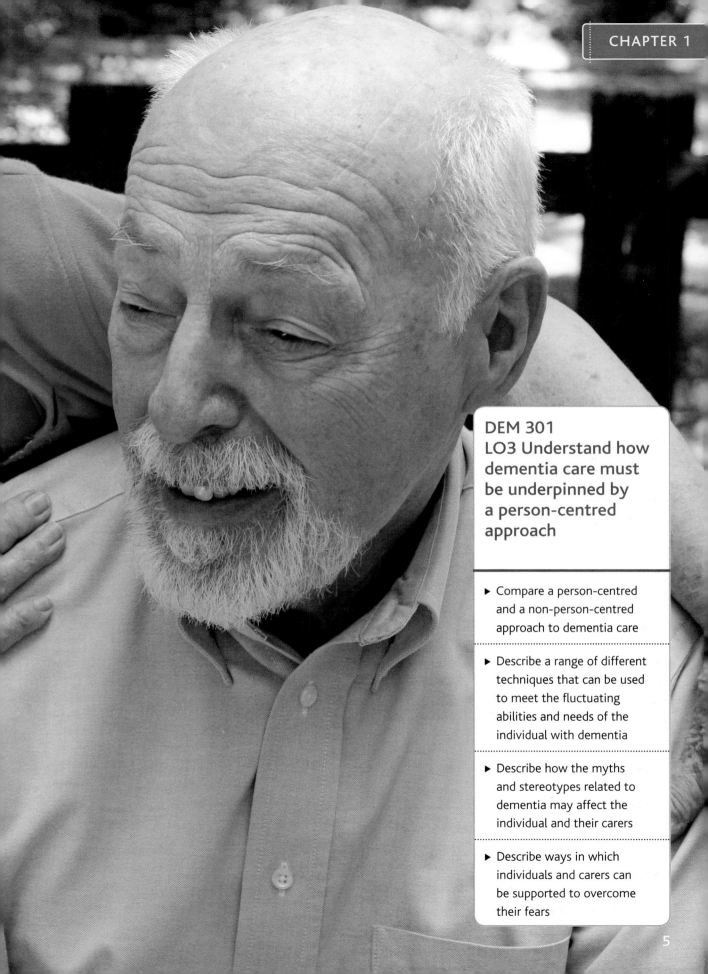

CHAPTER 1

**DEM 301
LO3 Understand how dementia care must be underpinned by a person-centred approach**

▶ Compare a person-centred and a non-person-centred approach to dementia care

▶ Describe a range of different techniques that can be used to meet the fluctuating abilities and needs of the individual with dementia

▶ Describe how the myths and stereotypes related to dementia may affect the individual and their carers

▶ Describe ways in which individuals and carers can be supported to overcome their fears

The neurology of dementia

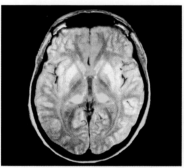

A brain scan can show changes in the brain caused by dementia

The causes of dementia syndrome

Dementia syndrome is a group of signs and symptoms that is characteristic of the condition. In dementia, irreversible changes occur in the brain of the individual leading to:

- death of nerve cells or loss of communication between nerve cells
- multiple cognitive deficits, including memory impairment
- problems with language
- failure to recognise people
- decline in overall mental function.

There can also be significant changes in the individual's personality and the way the person interacts in a social situation. Initially, individuals are able to care for themselves, but as the condition progresses the ability to self-care is affected, usually resulting in admission as an inpatient to a care organisation. Progression of the condition varies from one individual to another and depends on the type of dementia. Genes can play a role in some kinds of dementia, but the condition has not been linked to the inheritance of one particular gene.

Dementia syndrome covers the following diseases:

- Alzheimer's disease
- vascular dementia or multi-infarct dementia
- Pick's disease
- dementia with Lewy bodies (frontotemporal dementia)
- Creutzfeldt–Jakob Disease (CJD)
- Huntington's disease.

Key terms

Acetylcholine: *a neurotransmitter or chemical messenger that transmits impulses between nerve cells, including those in the brain*

Cognitive: *to do with thought processes*

Gene: *genetic coding in DNA that determines an inherited characteristic within an individual*

Hippocampus: *part of the brain that stores long-term memories of personal events*

Irreversible: *impossible to reverse or undo, as in a condition that cannot be improved*

Neurotransmitters: *chemicals that transmit impulses from nerve to nerve*

Stroke: *common name for the loss of brain function that occurs when the flow of blood to part of the brain is prevented, either by blockage or haemorrhage of a blood vessel*

Syndrome: *a set of signs and symptoms that is characteristic of a disease or condition*

Figure 1.1 describes the brain changes that occur for each of these diseases.

Figure 1.1 Brain changes occurring in different types of dementia

Type of dementia	Changes observed in the brain
Alzheimer's disease	Alzheimer's disease is one of the most common causes of dementia. It kills brain cells and nerves, causing changes in the chemistry and structure of the brain. The brain shrinks (atrophies) as the number of nerves gradually reduces. Brain chemicals (neurotransmitters) are reduced, in particular levels of acetylcholine fall. Gaps develop in the temporal lobe and in the hippocampus, both of which are responsible for storing and retrieving information. These gaps affect the individual's ability to remember, speak, think and make decisions.
Vascular dementia (multi-infarct dementia)	Tiny strokes (infarcts) occur within the small blood vessels of the brain; these are often so small that they are not recognised. However, oxygen supply to the brain is diminished and brain cells die. After each infarct brain tissue dies, so the individual's mental ability declines, eventually leaving him or her quite confused.
Dementia with Lewy bodies	Lewy bodies are distinct deposits of protein in the brain. These deposits damage brain cells and disrupt the brain's capacity to function normally, leading to degeneration of brain tissue and dementia.
Pick's disease	Damage occurs in the temporal and frontal lobes of the brain when individuals develop Pick bodies, another type of protein deposit. This disease is rare but has a genetic component and occurs in individuals below the age of 65.
Creutzfeldt–Jakob Disease (CJD)	Also known as 'Mad Cow Disease' because of the links between a variant form of CJD and a bovine degenerative brain condition. In all forms of CJD the brain develops holes and a sponge-like texture. This is caused by a protein called a prion, which is also an infectious particle. The build-up of these abnormal proteins spreads, causing nerve cells to die in the brain and spinal cord. The method of transmission is still the subject of research, but is thought to involve direct contact with infected material.
Huntington's disease	This is an inherited disease linked to defects in a single gene, which causes damage to nerve cells in areas of the brain called the basal ganglia and cerebral cortex. Damage to these parts of the brain affects the motor system.

Types of memory impairment

Mild memory loss, characterised by episodes of forgetfulness, is considered to be a part of the normal ageing process. However, for those with dementia, memory loss becomes a problem when it disrupts daily life. Several different types of memory impairment are experienced by individuals with dementia.

- A decline in memory function results in the loss of memories of recent events.

- Loss of memory means that the ability to communicate is reduced as individuals tend to ask the same question repeatedly, or lose the thread of the conversation.

- Problem-solving can become a major issue as individuals finds it increasingly difficult to learn new skills.

- Loss of skills is particularly noticeable, for example cooking, managing a household budget, remembering the rules of a familiar game.

- Intermittent moments of lucidity mean that certain abilities fluctuate, for example individuals may be able to hold a conversation for a very short time.

- Mobility can be affected as a result of short-term memory deficit; individuals can feel lost and wander away from their known surroundings.

Other signs and symptoms of dementia

Other characteristic signs and symptoms, in addition to memory problems, are movement difficulties – individuals can become unsteady on their feet and may develop a shuffling gait. Challenging behaviour may occur as a result of mood and personality changes. The individual can also become anxious, confused, suspicious or depressed.

Ways of enhancing the memory at early stages of dementia

Some individuals with early stages of dementia can manage well in their familiar home environment because they are used to where things are. Many also live with family members, spouses or partners, or have professional carers supporting them at home. Simple measures can therefore be used to enhance their memory in the early stages of dementia, such as ensuring a daily routine that includes reminders or written notes. These can inform the individual, for example:

- about when to get up and get dressed in the morning

Investigate

Using online and library sources, investigate the six different types of dementia shown in Figure 1.1. Try to find out which parts of the brain are affected by each disease.

Key term

***Memory impairment**: memory loss, partial or total*

- about when to put the rubbish out

- to remember to lock the door at night

- about specific objects that are used regularly, through labelling items such as mugs, kettle, television, cooker

- about when to go to bed.

Measures such as these can keep the memory active before dementia begins to disrupt the individual's life.

? Reflect

Identify an older person in your practice placement (or relative, friend or neighbour) who has dementia. Try to engage the person in conversation, perhaps asking about his or her experiences. Reflect on this and write 100 words about it.

Case study

Elizabeth is 70 years old and lives in Wales with her son, Joe. Until recently, Elizabeth has been coping well at home, even when Joe is at work during the day.

However, several times over the past few weeks, on returning home from work Joe has found Elizabeth wandering in the garden looking lost. When he questions her, Elizabeth does not know where she is and occasionally fails to recognise him. Once or twice Joe has found that Elizabeth has left the cooker on.

1. What symptoms is Elizabeth exhibiting?

2. Which type of dementia is Elizabeth probably experiencing?

3. Identify which part of the brain is affected.

4. Make a list of different types of memory impairment that Elizabeth may exhibit.

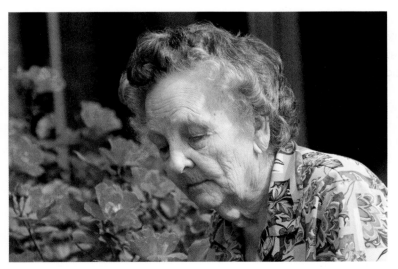

Memory impairment can make the person feel lost in familiar surroundings

Processing information

Individuals with dementia experience difficulties interpreting the world because of incorrect processing of information in the brain. This can result in significant problems with perception and communication, including the ability to articulate feelings. Frustration, stress and fear may result.

Processing visual information

The Thomas Pockington Trust (2005) suggests that there is increasing evidence of significant disturbances in visual function in Alzheimer's disease and other types of dementia. These deficits are believed to be more reflective of disturbances in the brain than of any problem with the eyes. Loss of vision profoundly affects communication. Problems with vision include loss of:

- visual acuity
- contrast sensitivity
- colour vision
- depth perception.

It has been suggested that hearing loss could be an early warning sign of dementia. It is known that the hearing loss in individuals with dementia exaggerates the effects of their poor cognitive function.

Memory

We all have two types of memory:

- short-term memories of events that have just occurred in the last few minutes
- long-term memory associated with past memories.

Individuals with dementia have short-term memory deficit and forget recent information, for example the date, time and year, or the fact that a relative who has just visited. Long-term memories, for example events from childhood, are normally recalled by those with dementia.

Information-processing problems

Individuals with dementia experience different information-processing problems depending on the type of dementia (see Figure 1.2).

🔑 | **Key terms**

Colour vision: ability to see in colour

Contrast sensitivity: ability to discern different light levels

Delusions: beliefs that cannot be challenged by reason

Depth perception: ability to see the world in three dimensions

Hallucinations: visions of things that do not exist

Visual acuity: clarity of vision

 | Investigate

Using online and library sources, investigate the way individuals with different forms of dementia process information. Summarise your findings in about 100 words and file as evidence.

Figure 1.2 Information-processing problems in different forms of dementia

Dementia-related disease	Difficulties in processing information
Alzheimer's disease	• disturbances in visual function, including impaired contrast sensitivity and depth perception • persistent and frequent difficulties recalling recent events
Vascular dementia	• hallucinations and delusions • blurred vision
Pick's disease	• limited attention span (easily distracted) • problems with sight and hearing
Dementia with Lewy bodies	• visual hallucinations of people and animals • spatial disorientation • difficulties with attention span • extreme confusion
Creutzfeldt–Jakob Disease	• impaired vision leading to blindness • other visual symptoms similar to Alzheimer's disease
Huntington's disease	• hallucinations • head-turning to replace eye movement

Factors that can cause changes in an individual's condition

Depression and other confused states are sometimes mistaken for dementia. This is because these conditions all have similar effects on a person's behaviour and communication skills. It is important to be able to distinguish these conditions; although there are notable similarities in the symptoms, there are also differences (see Figure 1.3).

Your assessment criteria:

DEM 301

1.4 Explain how other factors can cause changes in an individual's condition that may be attributable to dementia.

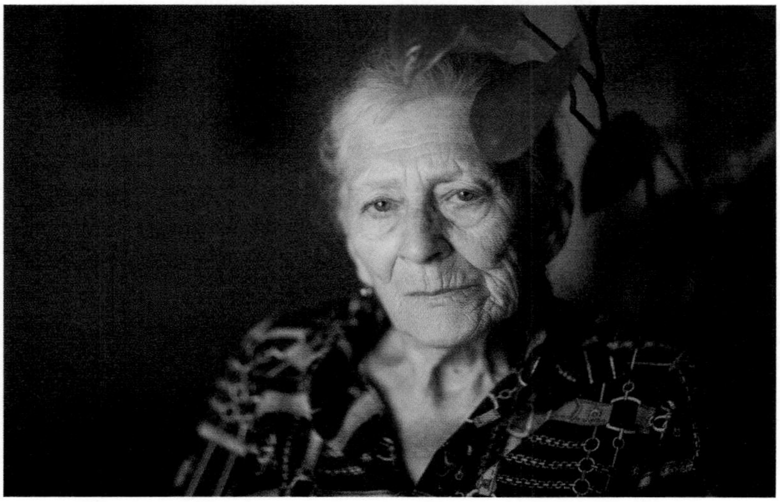

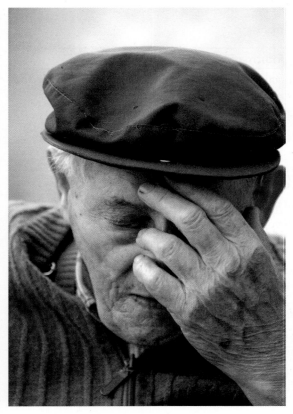
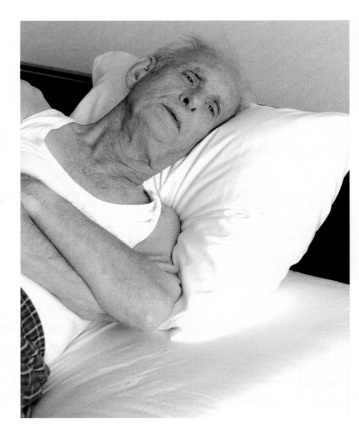

Depression is sometimes mistaken for dementia

Figure 1.3 The key differences between dementia, depression and confusional states

	Dementia	Depression	Confusional states
Mental performance	slow decline	rapid decline	temporary mental incoherence
Awareness of surroundings	poor recognition of familiar surroundings	intact awareness of surroundings	disorientated
Confusion	progressive confusion and disorientation	not confused but possible memory problems	confusion with difficulty in maintaining concentration
Motor skills	impaired motor skills including loss of the ability to write and even speak	slow speech and movement	
Memory	short-term memory loss, including specific problems with time	no short-term memory loss	poor short-term memory but improves when confusion passes
Other		a negative view of life	

Other conditions that may cause sensory changes

Be aware that there are other conditions that can cause sensory changes in the individual. These may not be attributable to dementia and could lead to a false diagnosis. Alternatively, they may present in an individual alongside dementia. These include:

- visual problems caused by age-related macular degeneration, cataracts and glaucoma
- age-related loss of hearing
- tinnitus, which can affect hearing and balance
- reduced metabolism causing poor appetite
- osteoporosis and fear of falling.

All these conditions can have a tremendous impact on the extent to which an individual is able to carry out the activities of daily living, depending on the severity of the condition and the person's ability to adapt and manage the condition. These factors must be taken into account when conducting a holistic assessment of a person to ensure that the individual is not wrongly diagnosed with dementia.

Key terms

Cataract: *opaqueness of the lens of the eye*

Glaucoma: *increased pressure within the eye*

Osteoporosis: *thinning of the bones*

Reduced metabolism: *slowing of bodily processes, attributable to an underproduction of thyroxin in the thyroid gland*

Tinnitus: *ringing in the ears*

Case study

Pam, 65 years old, has just retired from her job as a nurse practitioner. She led a busy life until recently; now she is more or less confined to her home. She lives alone in an isolated, rural spot, a long way from her family, but has a few close friends nearby. Her job kept her busy and also gave her an active social life. Now Pam stays in bed, refuses to do anything, has a poor appetite, feels hopeless and can see no future. Stephanie, a friend who visits weekly, has become concerned and has taken Pam to see her GP.

1. Can you describe Pam's symptoms
2. What do you think is wrong with Pam?
3. How can Pam's GP help her with her problems?

The abilities and needs of an individual with dementia may fluctuate

Environmental factors

The abilities and needs of an individual with dementia may fluctuate in response to changes in the physical environment. One of the fundamental characteristics of the condition is the inability of individuals to interpret the world around them.

Your assessment criteria:

DEM 301

1.5 Explain why the abilities and needs of an individual with dementia may fluctuate.

It follows, therefore, that any change in the environment can have a damaging effect on the individual. The following changes may influence an individual's abilities and needs:

- moving house

- going into a care home

- going into hospital

- changes of personnel, such as a new carer

- death of a family member.

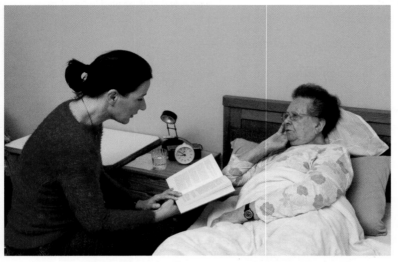

The care worker has an important role in helping the individual adjust to a new environment

Changes in the individual's condition

Other factors that may disrupt the course of the condition include:

- changes in treatment, such as taking part in a new treatment for memory problems

- changes in medication, such as taking new drugs

- changes in the individual's physical condition; for example urinary tract infections are common in older people and can have far-reaching effects

? | Reflect

Can you identify reasons why a person may feel very unsettled or even disabled by going into a hospital or a care home? Why might this undermine their self-care skills?

- vascular changes; for example transient ischemic attacks are temporary but are implicated in the development of some forms of dementia

- a change in the rapidity of progression of dementia, such that the individual suddenly becomes aggressive or agitated.

Emotional factors

Factors that affect the emotional wellbeing of the individual also influence the course of the condition.

- A change in the main carer, perhaps as a result of illness, can be upsetting, especially if the main carer is also the person's partner or close family member.

- Stressed carers may not support people with dementia to the best of their ability.

- The experience of any kind of abuse will have profound effects.

Key terms

Infection: situation where microorganisms proliferate inside the body

Transient ischemic attack: a temporary blockage in the blood supply to the brain caused by a blood clot and lasting about 10 minutes

Reflect

Can you think of anybody, perhaps a member of your family, a family friend or a resident in your practice placement, whose needs and abilities are fluctuating due to dementia? Why does this fluctuation occur, and how does it affect the carer? Keep your notes as evidence towards your assessment.

Knowledge Assessment Task

This assessment task covers DEM 301 1.1, 1.2, 1.3, 1.4, 1.5.

Dementia-based conditions are brain or neurological disorders. They affect the structure and functioning of an individual's brain and can affect people in a variety of different ways. It is helpful for both care practitioners and the relatives of individuals diagnosed with dementia to understand the neurology of the condition. In this assessment activity, you are asked to produce a poster or information leaflet that:

1. *describes a range of causes of dementia syndrome*

2. *describes the types of memory impairment commonly experienced by individuals with dementia*

3. *explains the way that individuals process information with reference to the abilities and limitations of individuals with dementia*

4. *explains how other factors can cause changes in an individual's condition that may not be attributable to dementia*

5. *explains why the abilities and needs of an individual with dementia may fluctuate.*

Keep the written work you produce for this activity as evidence towards your assessment.

The impact of recognition and diagnosis of dementia

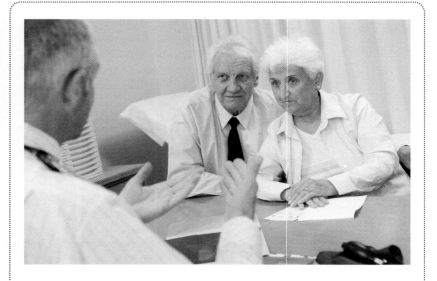

Benefits of an early diagnosis of dementia

Being given a diagnosis of dementia is a significant event for many individuals and their families; they may be aware that life is changing in a way that they cannot control. A diagnosis can create feelings of bereavement in individuals as they feel the loss of the person they once were. These profound emotions can obviously affect people's physical and emotional wellbeing, and their quality of life.

An alternative scenario is one in which having a diagnosis comes as a relief because individuals and their families have been fighting for recognition of a problem. Diagnosis may initiate access to services that they require. Even if receiving a diagnosis has a positive impact for some individuals, it may still be a difficult and emotional experience.

Figure 1.4, on pages 17 and 18, summarises the impact a diagnosis of dementia can have on an individual.

? Reflect

Do you think that it would ever be okay to keep a diagnosis of dementia from an individual experiencing the early stages of this condition? Are there benefits to doing so or is this an unethical and dishonest practice?

Figure 1.4 Aspects of an individual's life that may be affected by a diagnosis of dementia

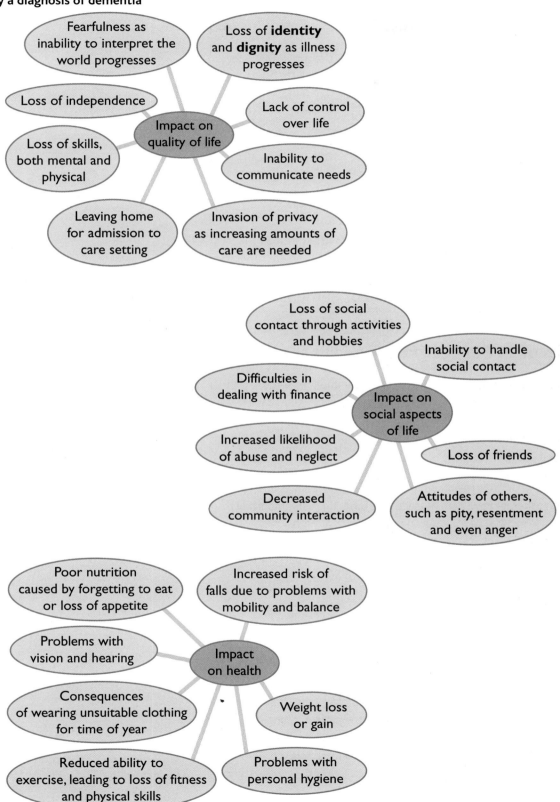

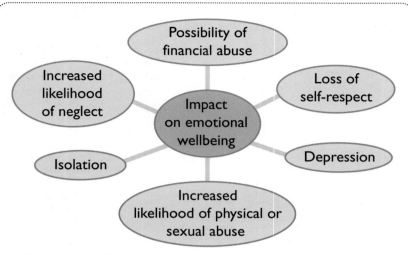

Figure 1.4 (continued) Aspects of an individual's life that may be affected by a diagnosis of dementia

Recording signs and symptoms of dementia

It is important to understand the reporting and recording systems in your organisation. Good record keeping is vital in providing care that is safe and effective. Increasingly, information technology and electronic record-keeping are being used, though it is still common for some records to be paper based.

Agreed ways of working

When recording possible signs and symptoms of dementia in an individual, it is important to adhere to the agreed policies of your organisation, whether in written or electronic form. It is very important:

- to record facts accurately

- to write legibly

- to date and sign the report

- to maintain confidentiality in line with recognised policies and procedures.

Recording changes in condition

It is important to record accurately not just the presence or absence of symptoms, but whether there is any change in the patient's condition, such as improvement or worsening of symptoms. This is could highlight a pattern in the progress of the disease. The Data Protection Act 1998 covers health records, and should be followed at all times.

Your assessment criteria:

DEM 301

2.2 Explain the importance of recording possible signs or symptoms of dementia in an individual in line with agreed ways of working.

 Investigate

Look at the records of one or two individuals with dementia who receive care in your work setting. Do the entries in their care records meet these criteria?

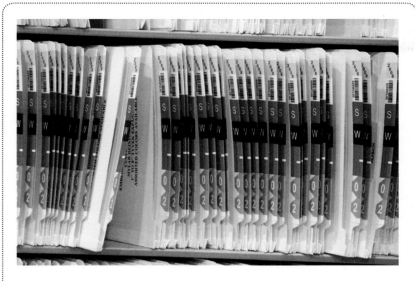

? | **Reflect**

Are you confident about your own record-keeping practice? Are there any aspects of this that you would like help or assistance with? Who could you approach about this?

 | **Investigate**

Ask the person in charge of your practice placement whether you can look at the reporting and recording systems used within the organisation. Make notes on the different systems.

Principles of good record-keeping

There are recognised principles of good record-keeping, which include:

- legibility

- authenticity – records should be dated, the time specified if appropriate, and signed

- accuracy – data should be factual, relevant and truthful

- completeness – full details of care and treatment should be included as appropriate and any identified risks should be specified

- compliance – records should adhere to any internal policies and procedures and to any relevant legislation such as the Data Protection Act

- protection – measures should be in place so that confidentiality is maintained

- originality – records must not be altered, destroyed or falsified; any necessary and permitted alterations must be signed and dated, and the original record should be clear and auditable.

The process of recording possible signs or symptoms of dementia

The process of reporting possible signs of dementia should follow the procedures used within your own organisation, whether these procedures are verbal, written or electronic.

The process of recording should also follow the principles of good record-keeping (see above).

Your assessment criteria:

DEM 301

2.3 Explain the process of reporting possible signs of dementia within agreed ways of working.

Case study

Hilda is an 87-year-old woman who has recently moved into a care home. She had been used to living on her own in a flat with her cat, but as her condition deteriorated Hilda reluctantly agreed to go into the home. From the start, the care staff noticed that Hilda was getting lost, and becoming quite hostile and aggressive with the other residents. It was obvious that she was feeling disorientated as she had moved from familiar surroundings to a very different environment. She was finding it difficult to settle and to communicate her feelings to staff.

An assessment was conducted on admission and daily records were maintained of her changing condition and worsening symptoms. The GP was notified of these changes.

1. Why is it important to maintain good records in the care environment?

2. What changes in Hilda's condition should be reported and what actions taken?

3. Suggest how care staff should ensure that the principles of good record-keeping are adhered to in the care environment.

The impact of a diagnosis of dementia

The person receiving a diagnosis of dementia may react in a number of different ways depending on the individual. There are mixed views about whether all individuals should be told about their condition, as some may find the diagnosis very distressing. However, it is generally considered by GPs to be good practice to give a diagnosis because this helps with planning for the future and with understanding what is happening.

Responses to a diagnosis can include:

- fear – of losing one's home, friends, dignity and privacy, for example

- shock

- denial of the disease by refusing to acknowledge problems

- a need for more information – about the condition, symptoms, treatments and long-term outcome

- a need for emotional support

- a need for financial assistance

- a need for practical support, from family and the statutory and voluntary services.

Your assessment criteria:

DEM 301

2.4 Describe the possible impact of receiving a diagnosis of dementia on the individual, their family and friends.

Impact on others

As well as the impact of the diagnosis on the individual, there is also a significant effect on the caregiver, family and friends.

Anticipating the behavioural and psychological effects of the disease can be a severe source of stress for the carer. Studies have shown that psychiatric symptoms due to distress are common among caregivers, with family caregivers demonstrating more distress than professional caregivers regarding the delusions, depression and agitation of individual sufferers. There is a strong relationship between the severity of disturbed behaviours and the distress of the caregiver (Lay Ling Tan *et al*, 2005). Possible responses of family and friends to a diagnosis are similar to those of the individual receiving the diagnosis:

- shock and fear

- denial

- need for information

- need for support.

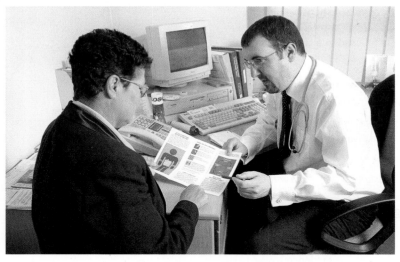

Giving a diagnosis to an individual needs to be handled with sensitivity

Investigate

Are there any dementia support groups for individuals and families affected by dementia in your area? How might these groups help people affected come to terms with a dementia diagnosis?

Case study

Brian is 79 years old and lives with his wife Lucy in a rural village. He lived an active life until about six months ago when Lucy noticed a change in his behaviour. He stopped wanting to go fishing and dropped his bridge class. He started to neglect his personal hygiene and seemed to be becoming increasing forgetful. He even got lost once on his way home from the library. Lucy has made an appointment for them to see Brian's GP together. Lucy is secretly wondering if Brian has Alzheimer's disease; she would like a diagnosis of his condition so she knows what is going on.

1. Do you think Brian has the right to know if he has Alzheimer's disease?

2. How do you think the diagnosis might affect him?

3. How would Brian's diagnosis of Alzheimer's disease affect Lucy?

4. How could Brian and Lucy be supported?

Knowledge Assessment Task

This assessment task covers DEM 301 2.1, 2.2, 2.3, 2.4.

Dementia is a condition that many people fear. Individuals, or their relatives, who suspect they have the symptoms of a dementia-related condition can respond in a variety of ways. In this assessment activity you are required to produce a handout that could be used in a teaching session for new care workers or students. Your handout needs to:

1. *describe the impact of early diagnosis and follow-up to diagnosis of dementia-related conditions*

2. *explain the importance of recording possible signs or symptoms of dementia in an individual in line with agreed ways of working in your care setting*

3. *explain the process of reporting possible signs of dementia within agreed ways of working in your care setting*

4. *describe the possible impact of receiving a diagnosis of dementia on the individual, the family and friends.*

Keep the written work you produce for this activity as evidence towards your assessment.

Dementia care must be underpinned by a person-centred approach

Two different models of care

There are two models of care: the person-centred or **holistic approach** and the non-person-centred or **biomedical approach**.

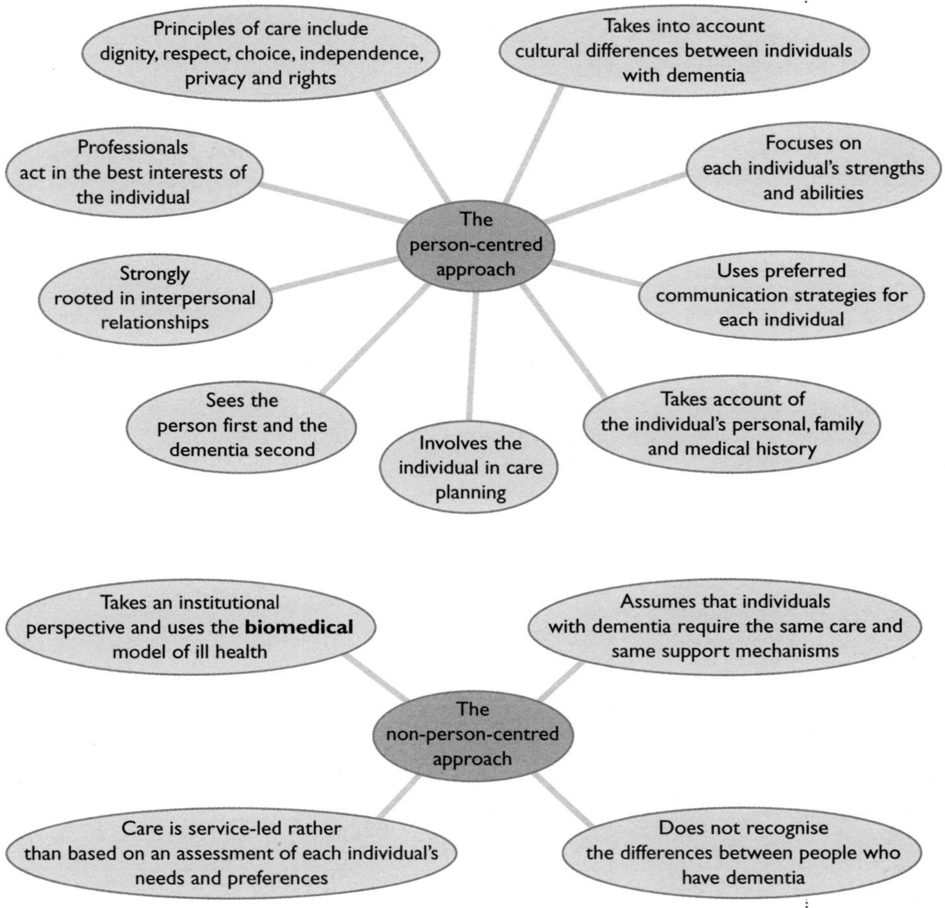

Your assessment criteria:

DEM 301

3.1 Compare a person-centred and a non-person-centred approach to dementia care.

The person-centred approach:
- Principles of care include dignity, respect, choice, independence, privacy and rights
- Takes into account cultural differences between individuals with dementia
- Professionals act in the best interests of the individual
- Focuses on each individual's strengths and abilities
- Strongly rooted in interpersonal relationships
- Uses preferred communication strategies for each individual
- Sees the person first and the dementia second
- Involves the individual in care planning
- Takes account of the individual's personal, family and medical history

The non-person-centred approach:
- Takes an institutional perspective and uses the **biomedical** model of ill health
- Assumes that individuals with dementia require the same care and same support mechanisms
- Care is service-led rather than based on an assessment of each individual's needs and preferences
- Does not recognise the differences between people who have dementia

Figure 1.5 A comparison of the person-centred (holistic) approach and the non-person-centred (biomedical) approach

Key terms

Biomedical approach: medical model of care that addresses the biological aspects of the condition, the opposite of the holistic approach

Holistic approach: person-centred care or care that focuses on the wellbeing of the whole person, not on treating the condition in isolation

Techniques to meet the fluctuating abilities and needs of the individual

Your assessment criteria:

DEM 301

3.2 Describe a range of different techniques that can be used to meet the fluctuating abilities and needs of the individual with dementia.

Two different techniques are often used to meet the fluctuating abilities and needs of individuals with dementia:

- reality-orientation approach

- validation approach.

Reality-orientation approach

Reality orientation is used to stimulate the memory of an individual with dementia and to facilitate orientation to the day of week, time, date, and even weather. This aim is to keep the person in touch with reality and the present day. Carers use tools to remind individuals of their current life:

- recent family photos

- flash cards

- a frequently changing display board giving the day of the week, time of day, date and year.

Investigate

Using online and library sources, investigate validation therapy and the reality-orientation approach. Summarise your findings in about 100 words and file as evidence.

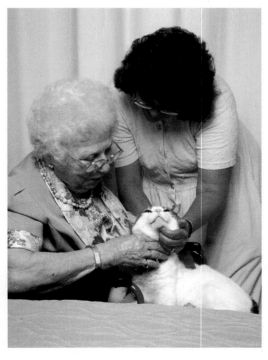

Validation approach

Naomi Feil developed validation therapy. It is based on a therapeutic conversation between the carer and the person with dementia. Whatever is

Investigate

Is a reality-orientation or validation approach used in your work setting to meet the fluctuating abilities and needs of individuals with dementia? Find out from a senior colleague or reflect on your role in the use of these approaches.

happening in the here and now, the conversation is based on past events in that person's life; this is especially useful if the individual has a limited recent memory. The positive interaction encourages the individual to take control of the conversation, and the therapy validates his or her feelings and emotions. The following are some tips for using this approach.

- Try to understand why the individual behaves in a certain way in response to a particular trigger. Try to get to the root of the problem by using a therapeutic conversation about past events.

- Individuals with dementia may not be easy to understand when they try to communicate, but they may still express emotions, for example by being tearful. These emotions are valid, so accept them even if the message is incoherent.

- Respond to what individuals say in a positive and encouraging way, even if you know that the events being described come from the distant past, or are not true at all. For example, the individual may talk about getting married. Offer congratulations rather than try to correct the comments.

- Ask specific questions during the conversation about feelings, and validate the individual's responses by expressing your understanding. You could say, 'I would be upset, too, if that happened to me.'

Using the physical environment

Assistive technologies can be used to meet the individual's fluctuating abilities and needs. The following can all be used to help keep someone with dementia safe:

- pressure mats that detect when a person is treading on them

- door alarms

- key pads on doors

- personal alarms

- handrails, non-slip flooring, bathing aids and walking aids.

Using the social environment

The social environment can be used to encourage positive interactions with individuals with dementia. Effective techniques tend to form part of a holistic, responsive and flexible approach, and include:

- reminiscence about past events

- involvement of family and friends

Investigate

Using online and library sources, investigate information on assistive technologies and the use of CAM in treating individuals with dementia. Summarise your findings in about 200 words and file as evidence.

? Reflect

Some people see validation as the kindest approach to use when a person with dementia is confused or distressed. Others see this as deceiving the person. What are your views on this?

Key term

Reminiscence: recollection of past events in one's life

- appreciation of the individual's personal beliefs
- a focus on strengths and abilities
- effective communication using preferred strategies
- appropriate exercise
- social activities such as music
- complementary and alternative therapies such as aromatherapy and massage.

Maintaining health and wellbeing

It is important to maintain the health and wellbeing of individuals with dementia by encouraging them to:

- eat well
- maintain their fluid intake
- exercise, for example taking daily walks or a gentle exercise programme that can be completed sitting in a chair
- engage in personal care, for example taking responsibility for their personal hygiene needs
- have regular checkups with a dentist
- have regular checkups with an optician and audiologist
- use both conventional and complementary medicines appropriately.

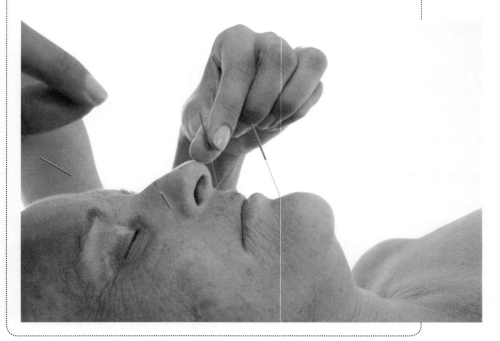

> **? | Reflect**
>
> *How do you ensure that the people for whom you provide care eat well and maintain sufficient fluid intake? Is there a way of reporting clients' eating and drinking problems?*

Using complementary and alternative therapies

Complementary and alternative medicine (CAM) covers a wide range of therapies that include:

- herbal medicine
- aromatherapy
- massage
- acupuncture.

A limited amount of research into the treatment of dementia with CAM has been completed. However, a number of therapies can be beneficial. There is evidence to show that both aromatherapy and massage reduce agitated behaviour for those with dementia, aiding relaxation.

Ensuring safety

Although most CAM therapies have a good safety profile, it is not true that they are completely safe. For example, there are concerns regarding some herbal preparations that may interact with conventional drugs. It is important for anyone caring for someone with dementia to check with a doctor before recommending any of these therapies.

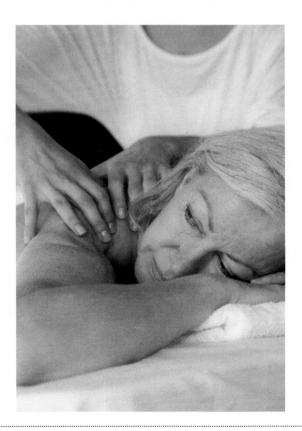

 Key terms

Acupuncture: *therapy using fine needles at specific points on the body to restore function by unblocking energy pathways*

Aromatherapy: *use of essential oils for therapeutic purposes, especially relaxation*

Audiologist: *professional who assesses hearing and advises on hearing problems*

Complementary and alternative medicine (CAM): *a group of interventions not considered to be part of conventional medicine*

Herbal medicine: *use of plants and plant extracts in the treatment of ill health*

Massage: *manipulation of the body tissue to aid healing or bring about relaxation*

 Investigate

Use an Internet search engine or other reference sources to find out more about complementary or alternative therapies that could be used in your work setting to help individuals with dementia.

Effects of myths and stereotypes

Myths and stereotypes can cause significant distress for individuals with dementia, their families and their carers. The stigma of dementia can negatively affect relationships with others, leading to social isolation for the individual, and possibly the family and the carer too.

There is often an assumption that, following a diagnosis, the individual will immediately lose independence. However, in the early stages of the disease many people with dementia are able to continue:

- making decisions about their own care
- driving a car
- caring for themselves
- communicating their needs.

Challenging myths and stereotypes

If myths and stereotypes are allowed to prevail, people with the early stages of dementia may avoid interacting with the medical community, leading to:

- delays in diagnosis
- lack of awareness of support services
- lack of knowledge about appropriate treatments.

Professionals who base their care on person-centred values should challenge myths and stereotypes by respecting the individual's rights, offering real choice, ensuring privacy, dignity, independence and autonomy. This approach is considered to be the essence of good practice and should be an integral part of the delivery of care.

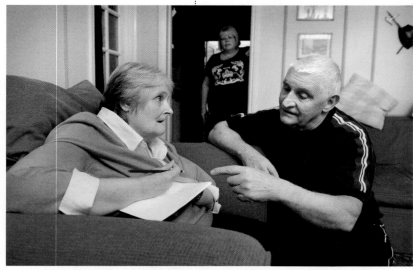

In early stages of dementia many individuals continue living with independence and autonomy, and carers can support them in sustaining this

Your assessment criteria:

DEM 301

3.3 Describe how myths and stereotypes related to dementia may affect the individual and their carers.

? Reflect

Reflect on the ways in which myths and stereotypes can affect the relationship between individuals and carers. Make notes of about 100 words and keep as evidence.

Overcoming fear

A person-centred approach that takes full account of an individual's needs and abilities can help address the individual's own fears and those of family and carers. When the best care, information and support are offered, fears generally subside. Individuals, families and carers can be assisted by:

- person-centred planning and case reviews, in which both the individual and the carer are fully involved

- involvement of the individual, family and carer in decision-making

- clear and accurate information about accessible and appropriate support services

- emotional support

- involvement with a support organisation such as the Alzheimer's Society, which works to improve quality of life for individuals with dementia

- an effective balance between protecting individuals and maintaining their rights.

Integrated service provision

Service provision should be integrated across private, statutory and third sectors.

- The private sector covers services that are provided by commercial and not-for-profit organisations.

- Statutory services are provided according to government legislation through the public sector (local authorities and primary care trusts). The role of statutory services is vital for people with dementia-related conditions. Increasingly, health and social care practitioners provide support for the families and carers of people affected by dementia too. This is important as it helps to maintain the individual's social support networks, and it can be the factor that enables individuals to continue living in their own home.

- Third-sector services complement statutory provision and are provided through voluntary organisations such as the Alzheimer's Society. Some specialist services provide drug and other treatments in specialist clinics for people showing early signs and symptoms of memory impairment, particularly Alzheimer's disease.

 Investigate

How do services for people with dementia work in your local area? Are they integrated so that there are good links and cooperation, or do different services work independently of each other?

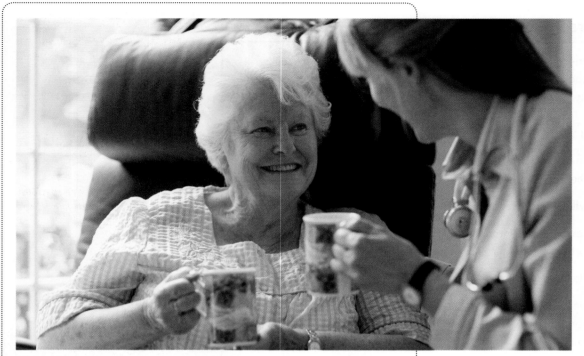

Individuals and carers can be supported to overcome their fears with help from a range of health and social care practitioners

Dementia Adviser Service

The Alzheimer's Society has developed a Dementia Adviser Service – volunteer and staff advisers support people with dementia, their carers and families through their experience of Alzheimer's. Access to a Dementia Adviser may help to allay fears. An adviser:

- is a named contact who develops a relationship with each family

- provides an impartial, high quality information and advice service

- focuses on individuals by empowering them to access the information they need

- collaborates with other health and care professionals, working in partnership

- enables those who are hard to reach to access appropriate services

- operates from a Dementia Adviser Centre that may be located in a memory clinic or GP centre.

Person-centred care and you

As someone with responsibility for dementia care, you can help individuals overcome their fears by providing person-centred care to the best of your ability. You can also help by being knowledgeable about the services that people with dementia can access. These include:

- hospitals and hospices
- residential care and nursing homes
- supported independent living
- sheltered housing
- day care
- domiciliary care
- GPs and pharmacists
- social services
- end-of-life support and urgent care response
- early intervention
- psychiatric services
- memory services
- physiotherapists, occupational therapists and dieticians
- other health and social care workers
- counsellors
- dementia advisers
- advocates.

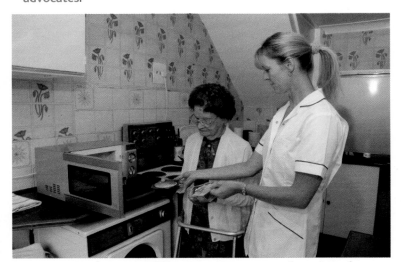

Person-centred care provides access to a range of services, from GPs and pharmacists to domestic help, supporting the individual through the experience of dementia

Case study

Frances and Fred have been happily married for 50 years. About 10 years ago Frances noticed a change in Fred's behaviour. Usually a patient and mild-mannered man, he was gradually becoming hostile and aggressive, with rapid changes in mood. One moment he would be happy and laughing, and the next very tearful. He seemed confused at times, finding it difficult to hold a conversation and unable to remember Frances's name. Fortunately, Frances was able to persuade Fred to see their GP. While conducting the assessment, Dr Long noticed significant memory loss and language difficulties. He informed Fred that he was going to refer him to the memory service for a specialist assessment.

1. Suggest how the memory service can help Fred.

2. Who will perform the assessment at the memory service?

3. What help and treatment could the statutory and voluntary sectors, for example social services and the Alzheimer's Society, offer Fred and Frances?

4. What other services could Fred and Frances access to help Fred live in the community for as long as possible?

5. How could CAM help Fred to feel less agitated?

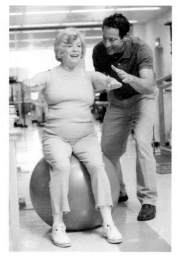

Overcoming one's fears requires the care practitioner to show compassion, respect and sensitive handling

Knowledge Assessment Task

This assessment task covers DEM 301 3.1, 3.2, 3.3, 3.4.

Compassionate, high quality dementia care is best delivered using a person-centred approach. This kind of approach may need explaining to new care practitioners and the relatives of individuals diagnosed with dementia. In this activity you are required to produce an information leaflet that:

1. *compares a person-centred and a non-person-centred approach to dementia care*

2. *describes a range of different techniques that can be used to meet the fluctuating abilities and needs of the individual with dementia*

3. *describes how the myths and stereotypes related to dementia may affect individuals and their carers*

4. *describes ways in which individuals and carers can be supported to overcome their fears.*

Keep the written work you produce for this activity as evidence towards your assessment.

Assessment checklist

The assessment of this unit is entirely knowledge-based (things that you need to know). The knowledge-based assessment criteria for DEM 301 are listed in the 'What you need to know' table below. In order to successfully complete the unit, you will be required to produce evidence of your knowledge of dementia, as shown in the table. Your tutor or assessor will help you to prepare for your assessment, and the tasks suggested in the chapter will help you to create the evidence that you need.

Assessment criteria	What you need to know	Assessment task
DEM 301		
1.1	Describe a range of causes of dementia syndrome	Page 15
1.2	Describe the types of memory impairment commonly experienced by individuals with dementia	Page 15
1.3	Explain the way that individuals process information with reference to the abilities and limitations of individuals with dementia	Page 15
1.4	Explain how other factors can cause changes in an individual's condition that may not be attributable to dementia	Page 15
1.5	Explain why the abilities and needs of an individual with dementia may fluctuate	Page 15
2.1	Describe the impact of early diagnosis and follow-up to diagnosis	Page 22
2.2	Explain the importance of recording possible signs or symptoms of dementia in an individual in line with agreed ways of working	Page 22
2.3	Explain the process of reporting possible signs of dementia within agreed ways of working	Page 22
2.4	Describe the possible impact of receiving a diagnosis of dementia on the individual, their family and friends	Page 22
3.1	Compare a person-centred and a non-person-centred approach to dementia care	Page 32
3.2	Describe a range of different techniques that can be used to meet the fluctuating abilities and needs of the individual with dementia	Page 32
3.3	Describe how the myths and stereotypes related to dementia may affect the individual and their carers	Page 32
3.4	Describe ways in which individuals and carers can be supported to overcome their fears	Page 32

2 | Communication and interaction with individuals who have dementia

**DEM 308
LO1 Understand that individuals with dementia may communicate in different ways**

- ▶ Explain how individuals with dementia may communicate through their behaviour
- ▶ Give examples of how carers and others may misinterpret communication
- ▶ Explain the importance of effective communication to an individual with dementia
- ▶ Describe how different forms of dementia may affect the way an individual communicates

**DEM 308
LO2 Understand the importance of positive interactions with individuals with dementia**

- ▶ Give examples of positive interactions with individuals who have dementia
- ▶ Explain how positive interactions with individuals who have dementia can contribute to their wellbeing
- ▶ Explain the importance of involving individuals with dementia in a range of activities
- ▶ Compare a reality-orientation approach to interactions with a validation approach

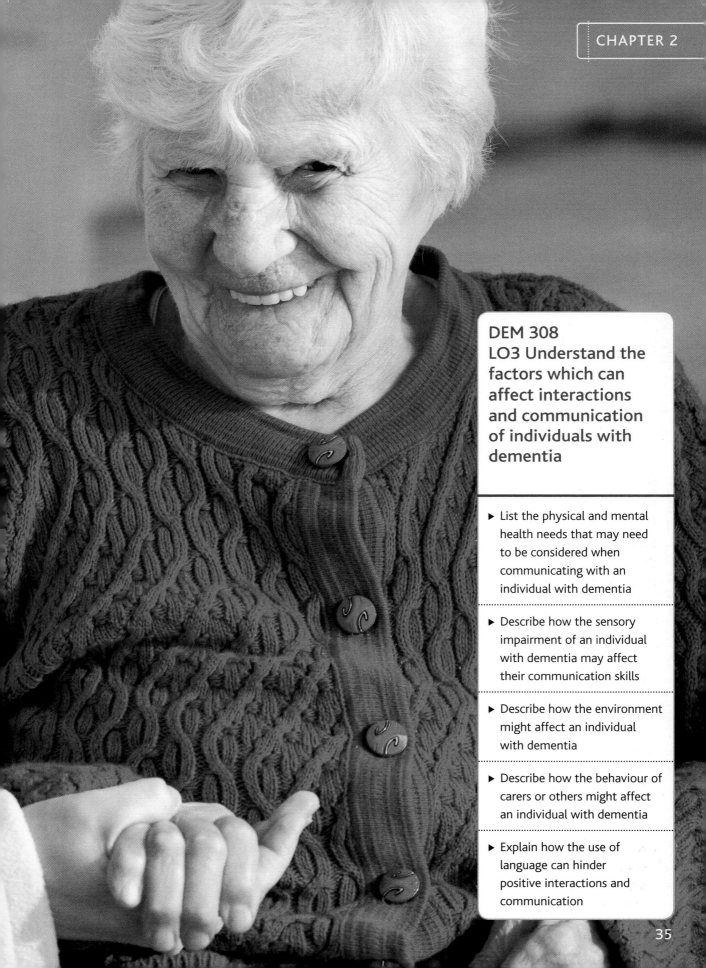

DEM 308
LO3 Understand the factors which can affect interactions and communication of individuals with dementia

▶ List the physical and mental health needs that may need to be considered when communicating with an individual with dementia

▶ Describe how the sensory impairment of an individual with dementia may affect their communication skills

▶ Describe how the environment might affect an individual with dementia

▶ Describe how the behaviour of carers or others might affect an individual with dementia

▶ Explain how the use of language can hinder positive interactions and communication

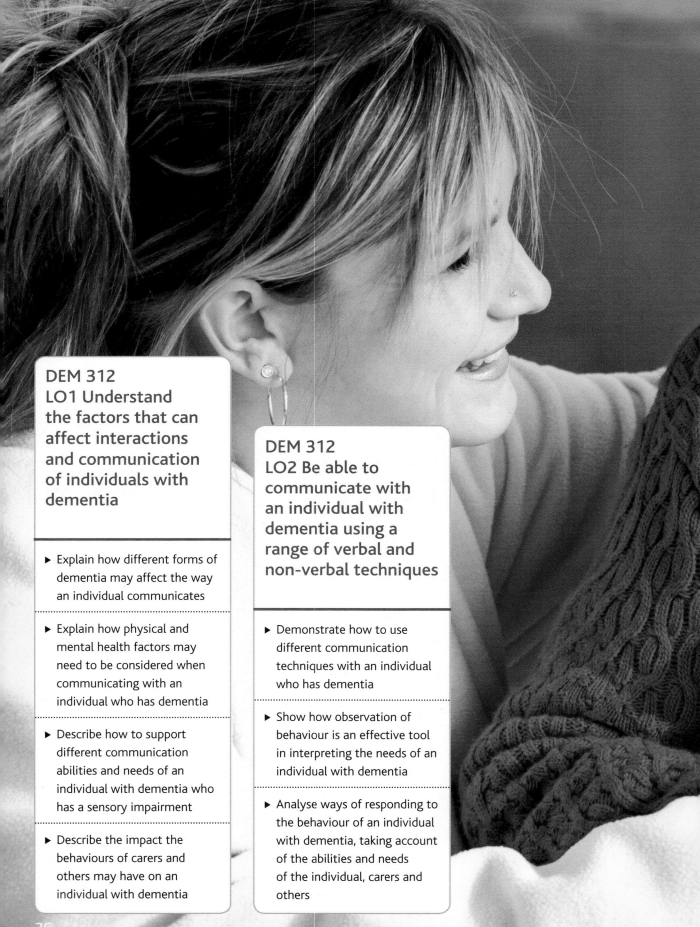

DEM 312
LO1 Understand the factors that can affect interactions and communication of individuals with dementia

- Explain how different forms of dementia may affect the way an individual communicates

- Explain how physical and mental health factors may need to be considered when communicating with an individual who has dementia

- Describe how to support different communication abilities and needs of an individual with dementia who has a sensory impairment

- Describe the impact the behaviours of carers and others may have on an individual with dementia

DEM 312
LO2 Be able to communicate with an individual with dementia using a range of verbal and non-verbal techniques

- Demonstrate how to use different communication techniques with an individual who has dementia

- Show how observation of behaviour is an effective tool in interpreting the needs of an individual with dementia

- Analyse ways of responding to the behaviour of an individual with dementia, taking account of the abilities and needs of the individual, carers and others

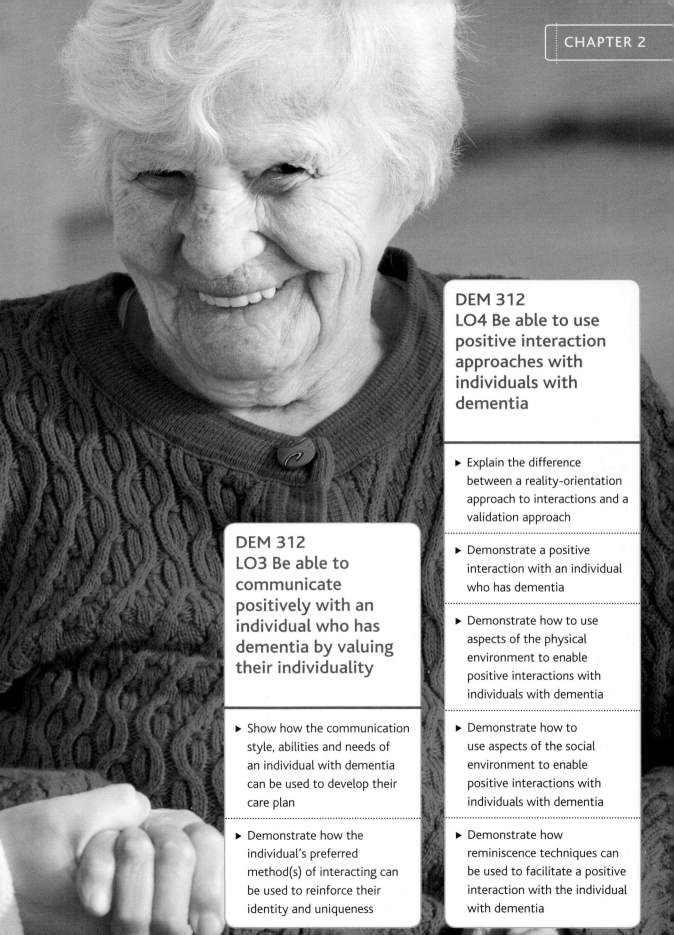

**DEM 312
LO4 Be able to use positive interaction approaches with individuals with dementia**

▶ Explain the difference between a reality-orientation approach to interactions and a validation approach

▶ Demonstrate a positive interaction with an individual who has dementia

▶ Demonstrate how to use aspects of the physical environment to enable positive interactions with individuals with dementia

▶ Demonstrate how to use aspects of the social environment to enable positive interactions with individuals with dementia

▶ Demonstrate how reminiscence techniques can be used to facilitate a positive interaction with the individual with dementia

**DEM 312
LO3 Be able to communicate positively with an individual who has dementia by valuing their individuality**

▶ Show how the communication style, abilities and needs of an individual with dementia can be used to develop their care plan

▶ Demonstrate how the individual's preferred method(s) of interacting can be used to reinforce their identity and uniqueness

How dementia and related factors affect communication

Introduction to this chapter

Interaction and communication skills are vital to our lives. However, interacting and communicating with an individual who has dementia requires specialist knowledge and skills. This chapter focuses on what you need to know and be able to do in order to communicate effectively with individuals who have dementia.

The chapter covers two closely related units: DEM 308 *Understand the role of communication and interactions with individuals who have dementia* and DEM 312 *Understand and enable interaction and communication with individuals who have dementia*.

Your assessment criteria:

DEM 308

1.4 Describe how different forms of dementia may affect the way an individual communicates.

DEM 312

1.1 Explain how different forms of dementia may affect the way an individual communicates.

Different types of dementia affect communication in different ways. In addition, physical and mental health conditions can have an impact on the ability of individuals to communicate and to understand the communication of others, especially where sensory impairment disrupts communication.

How different forms of dementia impact on communication

All forms of dementias share common features, but each is also associated with specific symptoms. Some of these symptoms impact on the ways in which a person communicates and understands the communication of others. Also, a person may have more than one form of dementia, such as Alzheimer's disease along with vascular dementia. Look at the table opposite (Figure 2.1), which identifies features of each type of dementia that affect communication.

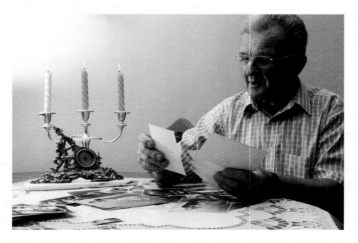

Key terms

Contrast sensitivity: ability to discern different light levels

Delusion: fixed belief that does not fit with reality

Depth perception: ability to see the world in three dimensions

Hallucination: disturbance of perception to one or more of the senses

Motion blindness: disorder of perception where individuals cannot see where they are going because movement is perceived as a series of still frames

Visual acuity: clarity of vision

Investigate

Using work, online and library sources, find out where the frontal and temporal lobes of the brain are located and investigate how damage to these affects communication for an individual.

Figure 2.1 Impact of different forms of dementia on communication

Form of dementia	Impact on communication
Alzheimer's disease: protein 'plaques' and 'tangles' develop in the structure of the brain, leading to brain cell death and a shortage of message-transmitting chemicals	Confusion; poor short-term memory – forgetting names/places/recent events Mood swings; feeling sad/angry/scared/frustrated but lacking words to express these emotions in socially acceptable ways, instead acting out through challenging behaviour Withdrawal and isolation due to communication problems Inability to follow verbal or written instructions; difficulty carrying out everyday activities Disturbances in visual function: impaired depth perception; loss of contrast sensitivity; poor visual acuity; loss of colour vision; motion blindness
Vascular dementia: a group of dementias caused by an interruption to blood flow to the brain	Symptoms remain constant, then suddenly deteriorate, known as a 'stepped' progression Problems with reduced speed of thinking, concentration Disturbances in visual function similar to Alzheimer's disease Hallucinations; delusions including paranoia (individuals believe someone intends to harm them and cannot be convinced otherwise) Increased restlessness; becoming obsessive
Dementia with Lewy Bodies (DLB): protein deposits in nerve cells disrupt normal brain functioning	Fluctuating abilities even within a day Spatial awareness problems – not knowing where their body is in relation to objects and other people Sleep disturbance: restlessness nightmares; hallucinations Problems with attention span/alertness; day sleeping – not awake when most people available to communicate Executive functioning difficulties: problems planning ahead and coordinating mental activities Loss of facial expression; changes in strength/tone of voice, making it difficult to interpret mood Extreme visual hallucinations, often of people or animals
Fronto-temporal dementia (such as Pick's disease): damage to the frontal and/or temporal lobes, responsible for behaviour, emotional responses and language	Lack of insight; lack of ability to empathise, appearing selfish/unfeeling Personality changes: becoming extrovert or withdrawn Inappropriate behaviour: rude/tactless comments; aggression; disinhibition – exhibiting sexual behaviour in public Compulsive rituals: feeling compelled to carry out actions, regardless of convenience or safety Language difficulties: not finding right words; circumlocution (using many words to describe something simple)

The physical and mental health needs of people with dementia when communicating

You need to be aware of the physical and mental health factors that could affect the way a person with dementia communicates with you. If you sense that something is causing the individual discomfort, pain or emotional distress, you will need to investigate further.

Some common physical and mental health factors that may affect interactive and communication abilities are set out in the diagram below (Figure 2.2).

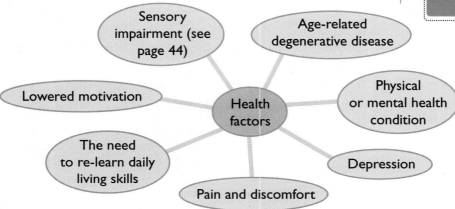

Figure 2.2 Physical and mental health problems that affect communication

Age-related degenerative disease

Most individuals with dementia will be in an older age group where degenerative diseases are likely; indeed, dementia is a degenerative condition. Other common ailments are osteoarthritis (wearing down of cartilage and bone in the joints), osteoporosis (bone thinning and weakening) and cardiac (heart) disease. Each condition brings a range of symptoms and reduced function, all of which can make a person irritable, tired and upset.

It is important for care practitioners to remain aware of the degenerative conditions a person has been diagnosed with, and to continue to provide necessary intervention and support. For example, if a person has been prescribed a splint for an arthritic wrist, the care worker should ensure it is worn even if the person forgets to do so.

Key terms

Advocate: person who represents and speaks on behalf of those who cannot speak for themselves

Degenerative disease: condition caused by wear and tear of the body, where the function or structure of body organs and tissue deteriorates over time

Also bear in mind that a person may have a degenerative condition that has not been formally diagnosed because of problems with communication. The care practitioner must act as an advocate for the person, passing on observations to a senior member of staff or a doctor.

Physical or mental health condition

There is a risk that the effects of dementia are so overwhelming that other medical or mental health diagnoses, pre-existing or a new conditions, can be overlooked, or symptoms can be attributed to dementia. The person may be unable to describe symptoms or give an accurate history of what is happening.

Where an underlying condition is known about, the person may forget to take medication, or overdose, and may forget appointments to check on progress, making the condition worse. Observation is a key tool for the care practitioner, who must notice signs and symptoms, recording and reporting these as appropriate.

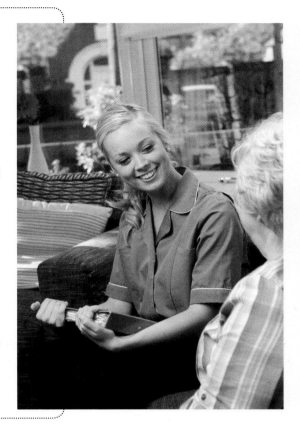

Case study

Patricia retired last year from her job as a district nurse. She has no immediate family, but her friends have always been important in her life. Now, instead of having more time to spend with them, she sees them less and less. An ex-nursing colleague and good friend, Georgina, calls round unexpectedly one afternoon and is surprised to find Patricia is in her dressing gown looking thin and dishevelled, with the house untidy and dirty. Patricia shuffles around holding onto furniture, and doesn't offer her friend a seat, or a cup of tea. When Georgina enquires whether Patricia is ill she denies it, saying she will be back at work next week. Georgina becomes really concerned and gently reminds Patricia that she has retired. Patricia looks stunned and begins to cry, shouting at her friend to leave the house and stop interfering in her life.

1. List the signs and symptoms of physical and mental ill-health that raise concerns.

2. What different conditions might Patricia be affected by?

3. What are the different ways in which Patricia's communication has changed?

 Investigate

Using work, library and internet sources, find out what various organisations, such as Alzheimer's Society, have to say about communication and dementia.

 Discuss

Talk together with colleagues about the different ways in which you can be an advocate for the older people with dementia who you work with.

? **Reflect**

Identify an individual within your practice placement and reflect on how physical and mental health factors affect his or her communication. Make notes in your journal.

Pain and discomfort

Pain and discomfort may be overlooked in individuals whose dementia makes it difficult to:

- recognise they are experiencing discomfort or pain

- work out the cause or source of pain or discomfort

- find the right words to communicate their experience

- answer questions accurately

- remember to take medication.

Again, observation on the part of care practitioners is crucial. For example, they should remain aware whether a person has been sitting too long and needs to be helped to move to avoid becoming stiff, or needs an extra layer of clothing to prevent him or her becoming cold. Behavioural changes that communicate pain and discomfort include:

- restlessness

- aggression

- frowning/grimacing

- rubbing/holding affected area

- screaming/crying.

Depression

Dementia and depression share some features. Some individuals with dementia are initially and mistakenly diagnosed with depression, and depression is commonly under-diagnosed in people with dementia.

Signs that a person with dementia may have depression are:

- appearing withdrawn/isolated

- showing feelings of worthlessness

- showing anxiety

- changes in appetite, including refusal of food or drink

- waking up early in the morning.

More severe forms of depression have symptoms more similar to dementia:

- memory problems

- slow speech/ movement

 Investigate

Using work, library and internet sources, find out about the incidence of depression in older people with dementia and the ways in which a diagnosis can be made.

- confusion
- a negative view of life.

The care practitioner must be aware of the behaviours that signal depression and encourage and support engagement. It is important to communicate empathy through words and actions and to maintain meaningful contact, as well as to report information to senior staff.

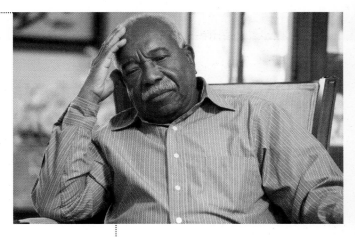

Lowered motivation

Individuals with dementia lose motivation and may appear lazy, apathetic and unwilling to do things they used to enjoy. They tend to withdraw from social and leisure activities, conscious that they cannot perform to their previous ability, and not wanting others to find out their illness is progressing. It is necessary for the care practitioner to keep people with dementia engaged and to ensure that communication channels remain open.

The need to re-learn daily living skills

Individuals with dementia often lose the ability to carry out many of the tasks that they used to be able to do without thinking. While individuals still have insight they may feel embarrassed and hide the evidence of their problems, such as telling you they have already washed or throwing away or hiding soiled clothing. Loss of skills may be particularly noticeable in relation to:

- personal hygiene
- domestic tasks such as cooking, cleaning, shopping
- managing a budget
- social conventions to do with communication, such as politeness
- taking part in hobbies/special interests.

As a care practitioner you will need to assess the person's daily living needs and provide intervention and support in ways that do not undermine further the person's confidence and sense of individuality. It will be important to:

- interact with empathy and encouragement
- develop a supportive relationship
- promote a sense of wellbeing.

 Key term

Empathy: ability to identify with and understand another person

 Discuss

Talk together with colleagues about the ways in which you demonstrate empathy towards the older people with dementia who you work with.

 Reflect

The brain damage caused by dementia can mean that simple tasks once carried out with ease, such as getting dressed, become very difficult. Try to consider how it might feel to be in this position and think about ways to communicate that support to a person and reduce their feelings of loss and frustration.

Sensory impairment and communication for individuals with dementia

We take in information about the world through our five senses. A sensory impairment interferes with a person's ability to accurately interpret an outside stimulus, whether it is visual, auditory (hearing), verbal, or through sense of touch or taste. This can lead to frustration, stress and fear if individuals perceive themselves to be in a threatening environment.

Look at the diagram below (Figure 2.3), which highlights some common sensory impairments that impact on communication.

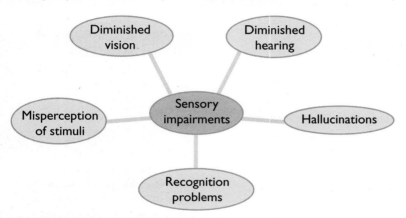

Figure 2.3 Sensory impairments that affect communication

Diminished vision

Vision is a key sense, and any impairment will have an impact on the individual's ability to communicate effectively: seeing the person we are talking to helps us understand conversation, especially by interpreting non-verbal communication (see pages 54–56).

A person with diminished vision may be short- or long-sighted, but may also suffer from an eye condition such as macular degeneration or cataracts.

Diminished hearing

Loss of hearing is another problem that may prevent an individual with dementia from engaging in interactions and communication. Hearing declines naturally with age, although some effects, such as a build-up of earwax, can be remedied with drops. Poor hearing affects speech recognition, reduces the individual's ability to attend to and respond to what is being said, and hence affects the ability to hold a conversation.

Your assessment criteria:

DEM 308

3.2 Describe how the sensory impairment of an individual with dementia may affect their communication skills.

DEM 312

1.3 Describe how to support different communication abilities and needs of an individual with dementia who has a sensory impairment.

Key terms

Cataract: *clouding of the lens of the eye, leading to blurred vision*

Macular degeneration: *deterioration of central vision, making it harder to see objects clearly*

Non-verbal communication: *way of communicating without speech, including conscious elements such as gestures and signs, and automatic responses such as posture and facial expression*

 Discuss

Talk together with colleagues about how it must feel to be deaf. You could even put ear-plugs in to experience something of this. Identify strategies to help when someone is trying to communicate with you.

Misperception of stimuli

Misperception occurs when information, whether visual or in the form of spoken words, is misinterpreted. Some visual misperception occurs as a direct result of damage to the brain from dementia. For example, a change in carpet colour between rooms, or a metal or wooden threshold strip, can be misinterpreted as a step, or a rug can be seen as a pool of water or a hole in the ground. Some individuals with dementia report a feeling of being lost in familiar surroundings due to motion blindness.

Allow plenty of time when helping a person to walk from place to place, making sure the way is clear of obstacles and that you provide appropriate support.

Hallucinations

Hallucinations can occur in all of the body's senses, including hearing, touch, smell, taste and perception of the body, but visual hallucinations are most commonly experienced by individuals with dementia. Visual hallucinations can involve seeing non-existent:

- flashing lights

- people

- distorted faces

- animals

- bizarre situations.

It does not help if you contradict a person who is experiencing hallucinations. Rather it is necessary to acknowledge the experience is real for him or her and to respond in a calm and reassuring way to help the person feel less confused and frightened.

Investigate

Try this experiment to give you an insight into some of the visual disturbances a person with dementia can experience. You will need a large, shallow cardboard box and a pair of binoculars. With the assistance of a colleague, look through the binoculars the wrong way, so everything appears further away, while trying to step into the box.

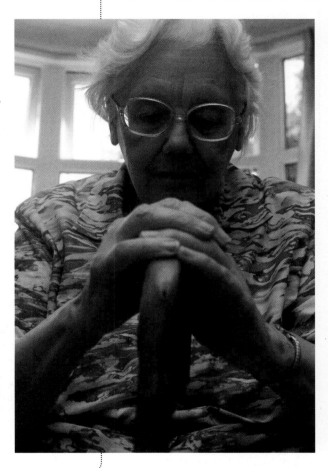

Reflect

Think about your senses and consider how these provide you with information about your environment. Consider, for example, the dangers of not being able to smell gas, or that food has gone off.

Recognition problems

A person with dementia may have problems recognising faces, even the most familiar ones, and also fail to recognise surroundings. This is known as agnosia. Even individuals with good eyesight can experience problems recognising what they see, and this can seriously hinder communication. Poor memory can play a part in this, but it is largely a feature of sensory impairment.

Allow individuals time to explore objects if they wish and give them information at a level they can make sense of. Sometimes clear labels on objects and signposts can help, including room signs with picture symbols or photos.

Support for sensory impairment

Hearing and sight should be assessed regularly, including when an individual is first admitted to a care setting. The checklist below (Figure 2.4) will help you with this.

? Reflect

Reflect on how you would communicate with an individual who has dementia and also hearing and sight problems. Make notes in your journal.

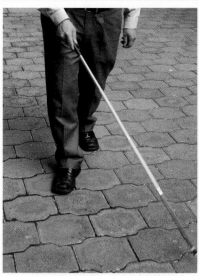

Figure 2.4 Sight and hearing checklist

Vision	Hearing
Check whether spectacles are prescribed and what they are used for, and remind the person to wear these	Check whether a hearing aid is prescribed and remind the person to wear it
Check the person is seen regularly by an optician who understands the impact of dementia	Check the person is seen regularly by an audiologist who understands the impact of dementia
Check spectacles are in good working order, and lenses are clean	Check hearing aids are in good working order, clean, and have working batteries
Check spectacles fit comfortably without rubbing on nose and ears	Check ears are clean with no evidence of soreness, inflammation or infection in or around the ear canal
Enhance vision by good lighting and keeping the area free from clutter	Keep background noise to a minimum (turn TV off; find a quiet room) when speaking
Use aids such as crockery with a band of colour to mark the edge of a plate; mark the edge of stairs with a line of contrasting colour; replace patterned carpets with plain; remove threshold strips between rooms; use large-print books and signs; provide talking books/newspapers	Use aids such as the loop system, and headsets for listening to TV; provide visual information

Case study

Dr Macy is 85 years old and a widower, with two grown-up children and four grandchildren who visit often. Tom's daughter, Beverley, has been noticing her father's increasing forgetfulness and he always asks her to repeat what she has just said, which she suspects is a way of stalling to give him more time to find an appropriate answer. He was well known for his wit and sense of humour and she finds it sad that he no longer seems to understand the jokes his grandsons tell him. In fact he doesn't even smile as much as he used to and prefers to keep to his own company.

1. What reasons might there be to explain Dr Macy's increasing isolation of himself from others?

2. What would you do if you were Beverley?

3. How would you support Beverley to communicate as effectively as possible with her father?

Key terms

Agnosia: inability to recognise what objects are or what they are meant for, or who people are

Audiologist: practitioner specialising in hearing and balance disorders

Loop system: device that enables deaf people to hear dialogue and sound in communal areas, by adjusting their hearing aids

Optician: practitioner specialising in eyesight and visual problems

Knowledge Assessment Task

This assessment task covers DEM 312 1.1, 1.2, 1.3 and DEM 308 1.4, 3.1, 3.2.

Different forms of dementia affect communication differently, and the impact of other physical and mental health factors must also be considered when communicating with a person with dementia. In addition, sensory impairment also affects communication and a person will require specific types of intervention to support communication needs and abilities. To complete this task you need to create an information booklet for new care practitioners about communicating with people who have dementia. Include in the information you provide:

1. *a description of the ways in which different forms of dementia affect a person's ability to communicate*

2. *an explanation of physical and mental health factors to consider when communicating with an individual with dementia*

3. *a description of the impact of sensory impairment on communication and ways to support individuals' communication abilities and needs.*

Keep the written work you produce for this activity as evidence towards your assessment. Your assessor may also want to ask you questions about the way you communicate with individuals with dementia in the work setting.

Discuss

Talk together with colleagues about the ways in which opticians and audiologists are able to assess the sight and hearing needs of a person, despite their being affected by dementia. Ask your manager if it is possible to arrange a talk with these practitioners to learn more about this specialist area of their practice.

Investigate

Using work, library and internet sources, find out information about agnosia and how this impacts on the life and experience of a person with dementia.

Supporting others to understand how dementia affects communication

Behaviour is one way of communicating. The behaviour of individuals with dementia can sometimes provide more information than spoken language, while at other times it can be difficult to make sense of. In addition, for a person with dementia the communication of those around them can be confusing and puzzling. The care practitioner needs to be aware of this and know how to respond appropriately, as well as supporting others to do the same.

The impact of other people's behaviour

Individuals with dementia may have a network of different people providing care and support. This includes family and friends, as well as professional practitioners such as care workers, nursing, medical and social service staff. People with dementia living independently in the community will also come across people through their daily activities, such as when shopping, while those who live in care homes will have contact with ancillary workers, such as cleaners, chefs and maintenance staff.

The way a person with dementia is treated by those who give direct care and by others can have a significant impact on wellbeing and self-esteem. The table below (Figure 2.5) shows the possible effect of certain behaviours.

Your assessment criteria:

DEM 312

1.4 Describe the impact the behaviours of carers and others may have on an individual with dementia.

DEM 308

1.1 Explain how individuals with dementia may communicate through their behaviour.

3.4 Describe how the behaviour of carers or others might affect an individual with dementia.

Key terms

Perseveration: *repetition of the same behaviour again and again*

Self-esteem: *sense of self-worth or personal value*

Figure 2.5 Impact of positive and negative behaviour

Positive behaviour	Self-perception in response to positive behaviour	Negative behaviour	Self-perception in response to negative behaviour
Being respectful	Valued	Being disrespectful	Worthless
Offering choice	Empowered	Offering no choice	Lacking control
Showing empathy	Understood	Being unsympathetic	Misunderstood
Offering support to make decisions within capacity	Listened to	Making decisions on a person's behalf	Unheard
Laughing with the person	Connected	Laughing at the person	Ridiculed
Encouraging as much independence as possible	Motivated	Doing everything for the person	Useless
Providing individualised care	Unique	Providing task-oriented care	Anonymous
Recognising and meeting needs	Safe and cared for	Failing to recognise or meet needs	Unsafe and uncared for
Acknowledging challenges the person faces	Recognised	Criticising a person	Humiliated

A person with dementia who is not treated in the positive ways outlined in Figure 2.5 is more likely to be:

- apathetic and unmotivated
- frustrated, aggressive and angry
- sad and withdrawn
- frightened, anxious and upset.

Changes in behaviour

Behaviour changes in people with dementia can be very upsetting for carers and family. The changes can be extreme and irrational. Typical behaviours include:

- **perseveration** (repetitive behaviour): repeating phrases and movements; repeated actions such as packing and unpacking a bag, continually asking to go home
- restlessness: pacing up and down, fidgeting
- shouting and screaming without an obvious trigger
- disinhibition: undressing in public or inappropriate sexual behaviour
- night-time wakefulness: turning night into day
- poor memory: asking the same question; forgetting things
- clingy behaviour: following loved ones or carers around the house
- interference: hiding and losing things; tampering with electrical items; making multiple phone calls
- suspicious behaviour: accusing people of stealing or tampering with their things, or attempting to harm them.

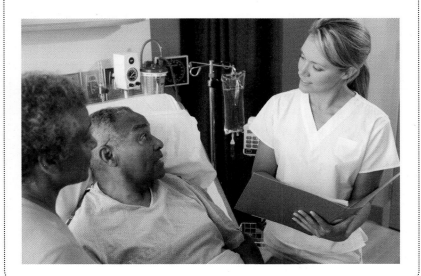

 Reflect

Think about a person with dementia who you know who has challenging behaviour and who you find difficult to support. Does it help if you try to imagine this person is a relative you are fond of, such as your granny? If you were to know more about this person's life before dementia, do you think this would help you to see them as a whole person and a unique individual?

Investigate

Using work, library and internet sources, find out about more about perseveration and the different ways this can occur for a person with dementia.

 Discuss

Talk together with colleagues about behaviours you have found challenging when working with older people with dementia. Discuss how you have coped and what you have found helpful.

Responding to an individual's behaviour

You can respond to an individual's behaviour both verbally and non-verbally. During verbal communication, you need to use a positive manner, and refrain from criticising or correcting the individual or carers. Non-verbally, you must show patience and understanding, because the individual and others will be able to sense any impatience.

You can respond to an expression of feelings either verbally or non-verbally. Sometimes the content of a message can be hard to understand; be sure to observe the individual's non-verbal communication to aid your understanding. Pay attention to:

- tone of voice
- facial expressions
- gestures
- other body language.

Using a sensitive approach, it may be possible to uncover the feelings the individual wishes to convey. You can respond by using appropriate physical contact to reassure the individual that you understand the situation; touch may be especially important if the individual becomes emotional. For some individuals, living in a care setting away from their loved ones can be very traumatic and they may require constant verbal and non-verbal reassurance.

Anticipating possible responses is very important; the individual's behaviour may indicate to you the need for help to accomplish a certain task; for example, individuals may fidget if they need the toilet or lick their lips if they are thirsty. You can anticipate their needs and offer appropriate help, in these cases assisting with toileting or offering a drink.

The care practitioner should engage with individuals, supporting them to make their own choices within the care setting, for example choosing a meal or what to wear. Time should be available for making these choices, so that the individual does not feel hurried or become agitated. A relaxed, unhurried approach is required and, if the individual has problems choosing, you should respond by finding out why the decision is difficult and by suggesting alternatives, if appropriate, in a positive and enabling manner.

Your assessment criteria:

DEM 312

2.3 Analyse ways of responding to the behaviour of an individual with dementia, taking account of the abilities and needs of the individual, carers and others.

? Reflect

Take time to observe the non-verbal behaviour of those around you and focus on the messages this contains. Also be aware of your own body-language and the way this could be giving messages you don't intend!

Investigate

Spend some time in your practice placement observing how your work colleagues respond to an individual with dementia and multiple needs. Describe how carers are involved in meeting the person's needs.

Misinterpreting communication

Being a carer to a person with dementia can be a difficult job. Sometimes the carer feels unsupported, unprepared and trapped in a role he or she never imagined. Some might feel they have lost the person they love to dementia, and when carers have little time to meet their own needs, this can lead to resentment. In this situation, it is easy for a carer to misinterpret the communications and behaviour of an individual with dementia.

As a care practitioner you need to support the carer as well as the person who receives care. You may also need to offer support to colleagues who find their role a challenge. It might be useful to share with them some insights about ways to think about challenging behaviours:

- All behaviour is a form of communication – what message is the person is trying to convey?

- The person lacks insight into their behaviour and cannot help it.

- Challenging behaviour is not deliberate, but a result of brain damage caused by dementia.

- Extreme negative emotion is often not meant to hurt, but reflects frustration.

- Shouting back will cause more extreme behaviour – a calm response is more likely to produce calm in a person.

- It is unwise to try too hard to help a person remember something that just happened, because it is not possible to recall a memory that hasn't been stored.

- There is a network of organisations and support groups that specialise in dementia.

- It is still possible to provide meaning and satisfaction in the person's life.

How you speak with and support carers will depend on their own ability to understand and act on your advice. Some carers are elderly and have their own physical and mental health problems to cope with.

The drawbacks of language when communicating

Dementia can make verbal language more difficult, both to produce and to understand, because it interferes with a person's ability to process information, remember it and express it accurately. The table on the next page (Figure 2.6) sets out the main difficulties that arise.

Your assessment criteria:

DEM 308

1.2 Give examples of how carers and others may misinterpret communication.

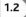

Discuss

Talk together with colleagues about poor practice you have witnessed with individuals with dementia. Why do you think this happened and what might have prevented it from happening?

Your assessment criteria:

DEM 308

3.5 Explain how the use of language can hinder positive interactions and communication.

Figure 2.6 Verbal language difficulties

Verbal language difficulty	Example
Chooses an incorrect word to express feelings	Saying 'tired' when meaning 'sad'
Can find only single words to express complex feelings	Saying 'worried', when in fact experiencing a mixture of anxiety, uncertainty, grief and a sense of loss
Talks fluently, but words do not appear to make sense (sometimes referred to as 'word salad')	'The talking microphone is table up and off'
Creates new words where the meaning is not clear	'Telebockteen'
Chooses words that are similar in meaning or sound to the intended word, but not accurate	Saying 'he's got a hairy' when commenting that someone has a beard, or stating 'he has a bread'
Repeats sounds and words that others say, but without understanding	Echoing what has been last heard
Loses the ability to start or follow a conversation	Unable to grasp the full meaning of what is said
Partially or fully misunderstands conversation	Not making connections and inaccurately interpreting what is said
Uses challenging or demeaning language, including swearing	'You're very fat/ugly'
Has a shortened concentration span; unable to focus for long enough to enable understanding	Unable to understand 'It's morning time so I'll help you get up and about now, ready to meet the new day', but more likely to understand 'I will help you to dress in your clothes' (while you point to clothes as a visual cue)
Loses the ability to speak a second language, returning to a first language	Speaking in a first language, but possibly able to repeat the information in English if prompted

Be aware of how you speak

As well as awareness of verbal language difficulties for a person with dementia, you must be aware of the things you say and how you say them, because this can also present difficulties for the individual. For example:

1. Do not to finish sentences for a person.

2. Do not ask too many questions.

3. Find out how to address each person, by first name or surname.

4. Do not use intimate terms of endearment, such as 'sweetie' or 'darling' unless you are sure they are welcome and appropriate.

5. Do not speak in an overly jolly manner, which can be patronising, or use a brusque tone that sounds dismissive.

6. Avoid using 'we' instead of 'you' (as in, 'Shall we get up?').

? | Reflect

Identify an individual with dementia from your practice placement and reflect on the impact the behaviour of carers and others has had on that person. Make notes in your journal.

Case study

Rita Day has vascular dementia and lives with her husband Eddie at home. Anshula, a dementia support worker, is visiting to assess whether more help is needed. Each time Anshula addresses Rita she notices that she looks to Eddie to give the answer, and when she does eventually reply he jumps in to finish her sentence or to contradict her. He even prompts her with the correct answers to questions that are part of the mini mental state assessment. While Eddie is making tea, Anshula comments, 'Mrs Day, you have a lovely home. Are those flowers from the garden?' Rita struggles to form her thoughts into sentences, but smiles and nods enthusiastically and appears to want to say more. Anshula rests her hand gently over Rita's hand, reassuring her that she can take her time. Rita eventually blurts out, 'I was a flower person – you know, in a shop. I'm so bad now – stupid. My Eddie fills in.'

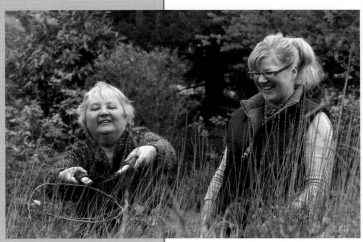

1. What do you think Rita might mean by her words?

2. How does Anshula demonstrate good practice in her communication skills?

3. How could Eddie improve his communication with his wife?

 Investigate

Using work, library and internet sources, find out more information about the relationship between types of disruption to language and the specific area of the brain that is affected by brain damage from dementia.

Knowledge Assessment Task

This assessment task covers DEM 312 1.4, 2.3 and DEM 308 1.1, 1.2, 3.4, 3.5.

Individuals with dementia can behave in challenging ways, and equally can be affected by the behaviour of carers towards them. Understanding what a person is trying to communicate through behaviour and responding appropriately makes a difference, especially with the knowledge that spoken language can hinder communication. To complete this task you need to produce a leaflet about communication aimed at carers who look after a relative with dementia at home. Make sure you include in this:

1. *the impact of carer behaviour on individuals with dementia*

2. *positive and negative ways to respond to the behaviour of an individual with dementia*

3. *what challenging behaviour might be trying to convey*

4. *how challenging behaviour can be misinterpreted*

5. *the drawbacks of verbal language.*

Keep the written work you produce for this activity as evidence towards your assessment. Your assessor may also want to ask you questions about the way you communicate with individuals with dementia in the work setting.

Effective communication techniques

Effective communication with individuals with dementia is important, and there are a number of useful communication techniques and approaches where close observation of behaviour is a tool in itself for interpreting needs.

The importance of effective communication

Finding ways to communicate with individuals who have dementia is important because otherwise they are likely to become isolated and withdrawn, which will lead to greater confusion and a further loss of their sense of self. Much of our human interaction and communication is complicated and subtle, and therefore difficult for a person with dementia to process as they once did. This means that to be effective communication must be clear, direct and simple. Others must be prepared to make time to listen to and observe the person, enabling his or her message to be conveyed successfully.

Using communication techniques

A number of techniques can be used to help individuals with communication difficulties to express themselves – verbally, or through non-verbal communication – and to understand communication. The table below (Figure 2.7) describes some commonly used techniques.

Your assessment criteria:

DEM 312

2.1 Demonstrate how to use different communication techniques with an individual who has dementia.

DEM 308

1.3 Explain the importance of effective communication to an individual with dementia.

Key term

Body language: *non-verbal communication*

Figure 2.7 Using communication techniques

Communication technique	Method
Provide a conducive environment to enable communication to take place	Position chairs at an angle, rather than side by side; this is more comfortable and less formal
	If the person is reluctant to talk, use a social situation, such as having a meal together, to create a more natural setting for conversation
Use non-verbal communication	Use a friendly tone of voice, smiling and nodding as appropriate
	Maintain positive eye-contact without staring
	Use touch appropriately to reassure the individual
Maximise understanding	Approach individuals from the front to avoid startling
	Face the person, speaking clearly and calmly
	Allow time and be patient
	Speak clearly using short sentences, and avoid overloading your message with unnecessary words
	Avoid expressions (such as 'getting out of bed on the wrong side') that can be misinterpreted

Communication technique	Method
Listen actively	Pay attention, show you are listening and take in what is being communicated, including through non-verbal information
	Focus on key words in the person's sentences to help you understand
Provide prompts	If the individual is in difficulty, make appropriate suggestions, checking you understand meaning
	Point to objects or people being discussed
	Use reality-orientation prompts, such as newspaper, calendar, clock
	Use reminiscence memorabilia
Use alternative languages	Use a sign language such as Makaton, which supplements spoken works with specific signs for objects and actions
Use appropriate aids	Use writing or drawing for messages if this is more effective than verbal communication (but remember dementia can mean that writing and drawing skills decline even before speech)
	Use communication boards and talking mats for the person to indicate feelings, needs or preferences (boards have been designed for specific situations, such as going to the doctor)

Non-verbal communication

Pay close attention to your own non-verbal communication and that of others. Sometimes, non-verbal clues may be the only indication that something is wrong, and effective use of your own non-verbal skills can help to draw this out.

Be aware also of body language messages you do not mean to convey, such as rolling your eyes, tutting and sighing while looking at your watch, which clearly indicates you are bored, or perhaps anxious about time and impatient to hurry away. Look at Figure 2.8 and the explanations that follow.

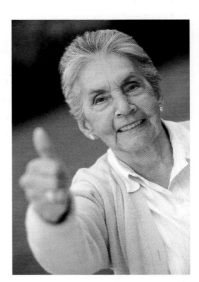

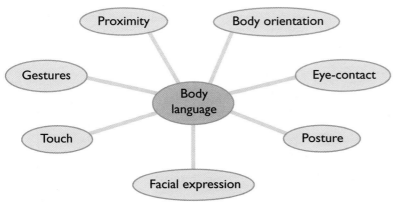

Figure 2.8 Elements of non-verbal communication

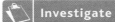 **Investigate**

Using work, library and internet sources find out about more about non-verbal communication and the power of body language when working with people with communication difficulties.

- *Proximity*: the distance between people. How close we stand or sit to a person relates to intimacy, and it can feel intimidating if a person invades your body space by getting too close.

- *Body orientation*: the direction of your body in relation to another person. If you stand squarely in front of a person, this can feel aggressive and confrontational; turning away might be seen as lack of interest.

- *Posture*: the stance of your body, which can reveal attitudes. Arms folded across your chest indicate a guarded, defensive posture.

- *Touch*: actions such as a pat to arm or shoulder and a gentle squeeze of a person's hand, used to provide reassurance and guidance. Use touch with sensitivity as some people do not like it and may interpret it as an invasion of privacy. Touch is also a safeguarding issue when you work with vulnerable people, and you must never impose yourself physically on anyone.

- *Gestures*: signs made with the hands and arms to illustrate or emphasise words, or to stand in place of words. People often gesticulate during conversations without thinking about it, but you can use gestures purposefully to make your meaning more clear. Be aware that gestures can have different meanings in other cultures. For example, a 'thumbs-up' gesture is a positive sign in the UK, but is an insult in Iran and other Middle Eastern areas.

- *Facial expressions*: expressions such as a grimace of pain, a grin of happiness, or a worried frown that reveal feelings. A blank facial expression makes it harder to interpret what is being said.

- *Eye-contact*: a person's gaze, which during conversation will move to and from another's face. Holding someone's gaze is a sign of intimacy, but to do so with a person you don't know well can make that person feel uncomfortable, even threatened.

Reflect

Think about a recent conversation you had with an individual with dementia. Reflect on the skills (verbal, non-verbal and active listening) you used to engage with the person.

Discuss this reflective account with a colleague. Arrange to be observed using your communication skills. Ask for feedback and keep this as a record of your skills.

Discuss

Talk together with colleagues about positive and negative uses of non-verbal communication with older people with dementia. Try some simple exercises with each other, such as gently covering your hand with another person's, or standing directly in front of a person in extremely close proximity.

Reflect

During your times spent working with older people with dementia, try to raise your awareness, particularly to listening and to watching. Notice how staff members speak as well as the content of what they say. Watch carefully and reflect on your own practice.

Knowledge Assessment Task

This assessment task covers DEM 308 1.3.

To complete this task you need to create a poster for display in the staff room of a care home about the importance of effective communication with individuals with dementia. Make sure you include:

1. *the reasons why a person with dementia relies on effective communication*

2. *what makes communication effective*.

Keep the written work you produce for this activity as evidence towards your assessment. Your assessor may also want to ask you questions about the way you communicate with individuals with dementia in the work setting.

Observation is an important tool for all care practitioners. What you notice can provide useful information to inform the care you provide for individuals with dementia. Figure 2.9 outlines a range of observations to be aware of.

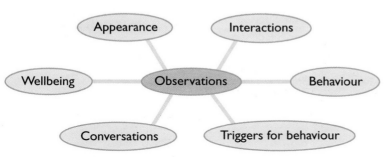

Figure 2.9 Observing individuals with dementia

Dementia care mapping

Dementia care mapping (DCM) is an approach used to observe, record and evaluate the experience and behaviour of individuals with dementia, as a way to improve the quality of care for each individual in a care setting. DCM involves observing an individual in great detail through a typical day. A 'mapper' can be an external person or someone from within the care team who takes on the role and shares observations with members of the team. This way of working can be embedded in everyday practice, and DCM feedback can help to develop an individualised and person-centred approach to care.

Your assessment criteria:

DEM 312

2.2 Show how observation of behaviour is an effective tool in interpreting the needs of an individual with dementia.

 Key term

Dementia care mapping (DCM): *technique used to observe an individual's experience and behaviour in the care setting*

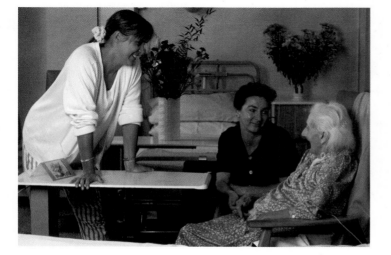

Dementia care mapping involves observing:

- how care is distributed among a group of individuals in a care setting

- how care was delivered to and received by an individual, including gathering feedback directly from the person

- whether an individualised programme of care is being used to meet the person's needs

- behaviours the individual is engaged in (for example, does the person become agitated or start undressing when in need of the toilet, or shout out or wander around when bored?)

- the style used by the practitioner when delivering care (for example, was it empathic and caring?)

- how the individual responds to particular practitioners

- whether the responses from the practitioners instil a sense of wellbeing

- whether the practitioners promote person-centred care and have positive interactions with the individual

- interactions with family members; this includes gathering their feedback.

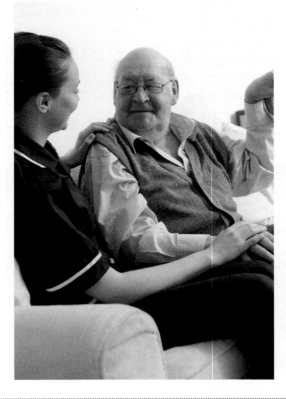

Investigate

Using online and library sources, investigate how Dementia Care Mapping is used in practice settings with individuals who have dementia.

- *Find out whether DCM is being used at your practice placement.*

- *Ask whether you can observe a DCM mapper and find out how this approach is applied in practice. Make notes about your findings.*

The difference between a reality-orientation and a validation approach

Two approaches to communication that are successful with individuals with dementia are a reality-orientation approach and a validation approach. It is possible to use elements of each approach with the same person, by using sensitive judgment to recognise which would be more appropriate and effective in the moment. Figure 2.10 highlights the key components of each approach.

Your assessment criteria:

DEM 312

4.1 Explain the difference between a reality-orientation approach to interactions and a validation approach.

DEM 308

2.4 Compare a reality-orientation approach to interactions with a validation approach.

Figure 2.10 Reality-orientated and validation approaches

Reality orientation	Validation therapy
Can be undertaken in groups or individually	Is undertaken at an individual level
Sets out to orientate the person in time and space, providing a foundation in reality for those unable to do this for themselves	Accepts at face value what a person says (which may not make sense or conform with reality)
Emphasises rehearsal of key information, where mistakes and misconceptions are corrected	Is not concerned with facts, but focuses on and relates to the feelings behind words, believing that forcing someone to accept aspects of reality that they cannot comprehend is unkind and psychologically damaging
Uses visual prompts, such as signs, clocks, calendars, diaries and notebooks	Empathises with a person's perceptions in order to achieve a better understanding of his or her behaviour
Aims at key information being retained, such as the location of toilet or bedroom	Explores an individual's own reality by asking who, what, where, when, and how
Never misinforms individuals, but constantly reorientates them to their present reality	Understands individuals are letting you know about their reality, which holds meaning for them and is therefore valid
Can help a person feel more secure and aware of the immediate surroundings	Accepts individuals as they are and validates a person's desire to communicate, using this to build a therapeutic relationship

Here is an example demonstrating how the two approaches can be used.

Sam worked in the same factory for 35 years and believes today is like any other weekday. He thinks that he must get his tools together and catch the works bus. The reality-orientation approach would gently and tactfully remind Sam that he retired five years ago and no longer needs to worry about getting ready or rushing for the bus. Emphasis may be placed on reminding Sam of where he is now, why he is there, and what activities he could be doing instead.

In contrast, the validation approach would not challenge Sam's belief in his job but would reassure him, perhaps, that there is no need to rush today. The care practitioner might encourage Sam to chat about his work and find out whether his belief that he is going to work reflects an inner

Key terms

Reality-orientation approach: technique used to facilitate orientation to the day of week, time, date, and even weather

Validation approach: therapeutic conversation with the individual based on past events

anxiety or excited anticipation about anything. The care practitioner could also suggest that, since he always works so hard, perhaps he deserves a day off, and steer him towards other activities.

Case study

Rosa, who is Spanish, has dementia and has lived in residential care for so many years she considers it home, even answering the doorbell and welcoming people in. She dances in the large hallway, clicking imaginary castanets in her hands. She tells anyone who wants to listen that she is a famous flamenco dancer and will be appearing at the concert hall next week. Maisie, the cleaner, always stops for a chat and often dances alongside Rosa or applauds her, saying 'Bravo!' and 'Encore!' Babs, a care practitioner, tells Maisie that she shouldn't go along with Rosa's ideas, because it only makes her worse. She gently reminds Rosa: 'You are in a care home now, but you used to teach English to Spanish people. I don't think you were ever a professional flamenco dancer.'

1. What different communication approaches are Maisie and Babs using, and what are the strengths of each?

2. On this occasion, which approach do you think is most successful?

3. Can you think of occasions when the other approach might be more appropriate?

Investigate

Using online and library sources, investigate the two approaches of reality-orientation and validation therapy. Makes notes on your findings.

Observe how the two approaches are used in your practice placement. Make notes following your observation.

Keep your notes as evidence towards assessment.

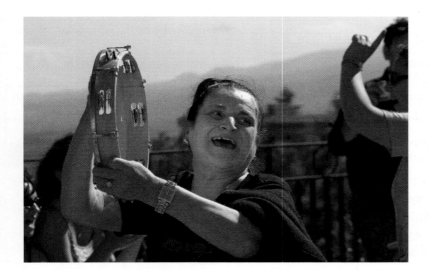

Knowledge Assessment Task

This assessment task covers DEM 312 4.1 and DEM 308 2.4.

The two approaches of reality-orientation and validation are both useful when communicating with a person with dementia; sometimes one is more relevant or effective in certain situations. To complete this task you need to:

1. *provide a short explanation of reality-orientation and validation approaches*

2. *read the short scenario below and answer the questions that follow.*

Chrissie regularly rattles the door of the care home, calling for help through the letterbox to passers-by, saying her children are at home on their own and she is locked in. She paces the corridor, wringing her hands and repeating, 'My poor babies. What will become of them?'

1. *Describe how you would respond to the situation using a reality-orientation approach.*

2. *Describe how you would respond to the situation using a validation approach.*

Keep the written work you produce for this activity as evidence towards your assessment. Your assessor may also want to ask you questions about the way you communicate with individuals with dementia in the work setting.

? Reflect

How would you respond to a person telling you that validation therapy is wrong, because it patronises another person, allowing them to continue to believe something that is untrue, like a child believing in fairies.

Practical Assessment Task

This assessment task covers DEM 312 2.1, 2.2.

A number of communication techniques use a range of verbal and non-verbal methods, as well as observation, in order to understand the communication of an individual with dementia. In this task you need to demonstrate through your practice that you can:

1. *use different communication techniques appropriately with an individual who has dementia*

2. *show how observation of behaviour is an effective tool in interpreting the needs of an individual with dementia.*

Your evidence must be based on your practice in a real work environment and must be witnessed by or be in a format acceptable to your assessor.

Acknowledging the unique individual

Each person with dementia is unique, so care planning must take into account individuals' communication style, abilities and needs, and reflect their preferred methods of interaction in ways that reinforce their identity.

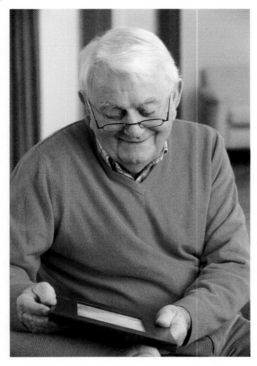

Your assessment criteria:

DEM 312

3.1 Show how the communication style, abilities and needs of an individual with dementia can be used to develop their care plan.

3.2 Demonstrate how the individual's preferred method(s) of interacting can be used to reinforce their identity and uniqueness.

Communication style, abilities and needs

The communication style of a person with dementia is the manner in which he or she tends to communicate. A person might be formal or casual, have a jokey sense of humour, be loud and expressive, or prefer quieter ways to communicate and interact with others. Some individuals may not speak, but perhaps their facial expression indicates that they are interested in what is going on, or perhaps they are warm and affectionate in their interactions, wanting to hold and kiss your hand.

As a health or social care practitioner you should be familiar with each individual's natural style of communication, mirroring this in your dealings with that person and including it in his or her care plan.

Individuals' ability to communicate (their strengths and competencies), as well as their communication needs (any deficits and areas requiring support) must also be taken into account when developing their care plans.

To ensure coordinated care between members of a health and social care team, you need to document in a care plan the communication strategies used to engage the individual and to create opportunities for further communication and interaction. The care-planning process should, as far as possible, involve the person, along with significant others such as partners, family members and close friends, as well as other members of the health and social care team. Communication strategies could include:

- use of memorabilia such as family photos and familiar objects that hold significance to the individual, reawakening dormant memories and helping a person to feel at home

- creating interest groups connected with a hobby, where communication flows during an activity

- creating social groups, where individuals meet to chat informally or reminisce over refreshments

- one-to-one sessions, perhaps building a life story together

- visits to places of interest, which stimulate conversations and interaction

- welcoming visitors, such as a church group or a person bringing in a pet.

There is more about this on pages 68–69.

Reflect

Consider how well you really know the older people with dementia who you work with. How familiar are you with their communication strengths and do you and other staff members play to these strengths to encourage further communication?

Key term

Memorabilia: *items that evoke memories*

Figure 2.11 Example care plan showing alternative communication strategies

Communication strengths and abilities	Planning	Implementation	Evaluation
Stan relates best in a one-to-one situation	Try regular one-to-one sessions	Key worker to coordinate a 10-minute one-to-one session every day	One-to-one sessions shared between three different staff members, working best when the cat sits on Stan's knee and he talks as he strokes it
Stan misses his dog and loves the pet cat at the care home, talking to it and stroking it	Arrange for Stan's dog to come to the care home	Stan's wife to be asked to bring dog to the home each Saturday afternoon	Stan was very emotional when his dog visited, but was clearly thrilled and asks every day if the dog will come

Preferred methods of interacting

Preferred methods of interacting will become clear as communication styles, abilities and needs are recognised and recorded in care plans. Health and social care practitioners should use these to inform and build their relationship with the individual, and through this process a clearer sense of each person as a unique individual should emerge. Indeed, this describes a person-centred approach to care.

One example is an individual with poor short-term, but good long-term memory, who may be helped to compile a life-story book, which can continue to be used by staff to help the person reminisce and to develop relationships. Similarly a person with dementia who retains a musical ability may be encouraged to play the piano, sing or listen to music as positive ways of interacting.

Life-story work

A life-story book is a method of working with a person to trace the course of his or her life from childhood and to record it. This can be done by compiling a scrapbook or album with photos and other mementoes, or it can be recorded through conversations. It is a useful method for interacting with an individual as it:

- provides an opportunity to build a relationship with the individual

- improves self-esteem by showing interest in the person and enabling him or her to demonstrate that long-term memory remains intact

- helps the person to recall significant milestones and express thoughts and feelings

- provides a tool for personal reminiscence, which is usually enjoyable

- draws in family and friends

- reinforces the individual's sense of identity and uniqueness.

Be aware that this method:

- needs commitment to make it work, as the process takes time

- involves personal and family information that needs to be handled sensitively

- brings up all sorts of information including facts, gossip and anecdotal evidence, religious and family stories

- might cause the individual to remember painful memories that stir emotion.

 Discuss

Talk together with colleagues about the care plans used where you work and how well these are designed and completed by staff members. Consider whether improvements could be made to capture the unique strengths and needs.

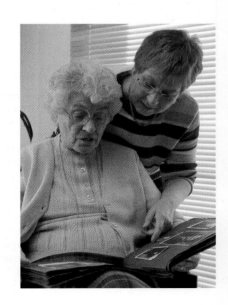

Case study

Rebecca is in the earlier stages of dementia and now lives in sheltered accommodation with her cat, Molly. She was once a music teacher and would still play a piano if she had room for one. She loves all sorts of music and plays CDs in preference to watching TV, saying sadly that she used to be knowledgeable about it, but can no longer remember facts. Her niece visits weekly, but Rebecca has few other social contacts and is rather isolated. She recognises her need to get out more, but doesn't feel confident on her own. At a recent assessment of need it was suggested she could attend a day centre twice a week, but she is reluctant to do this, fearing she won't remember people's names and that the activities on offer won't interest her.

1. How would you identify Rebecca's communication style, abilities and needs in a care plan?

2. How might Rebecca be convinced to attend the day centre?

3. Would life-story work help to develop a relationship with Rebecca, and how might you introduce and follow through this idea?

Investigate

Speak to your manager about encouraging the families and friends of older people with dementia who you work with to bring in items that can be used for reminiscence with their loved ones.

Practical Assessment Task

This assessment task covers DEM 312 3.1, 3.2.

Health and social care practitioners who work with individuals with dementia need to draw up a communication care plan that recognises different communication styles, identifies abilities and needs, and takes into account people's preferred method of communicating in order to acknowledge their unique identity. To complete this assessment you need to:

1. *identify an individual you work with who has dementia, and obtain his or her consent (speak with your manager/ assessor if this is not possible)*

2. *draw up a care plan based on the one shown in (Figure 2.11 on page 63).*

Your care plan should:

1. *include communication style; strengths and abilities; needs*

2. *detail how you will use family photos and other personal items to interact with the person*

3. *identify communication preferences*

4. *show involvement of others who communicate with the individual*

5. *reflect the unique identity of the individual.*

Your evidence must be based on your practice in a real work environment and must be witnessed by or be in a format acceptable to your assessor. Keep any written work you produce as evidence.

65

Enabling positive interaction

A positive interaction with a person with dementia can be described as any encounter, individually or in a group, that leaves the person feeling satisfied that he or she has been acknowledged as a unique person, listened to, understood and appreciated. Positive interactions can be achieved through activities that make use of the physical and social environment, and reminiscence is a key technique.

Ways to enable positive interactions

A number of considerations are important in enabling positive interactions to take place.

- *Enjoyment*: Before engaging in an activity, find out if the individual might enjoy it. Do not engage in an activity that individuals dislike, because they will probably lose interest. This means you must know something about individuals and what is likely to engage their interest.

- *Timing*: Choose a time of day when the person is most alert and awake and open to new stimulus. This means that planned activities timetabled into a regular weekly programme will not work for all people, because they do not take into account individual needs.

- *Personal comfort*: Individuals cannot relax and engage if they are too hot or too cold, hungry or too full, sleepy after a meal, or need to go to the toilet.

- *Preparation*: Make sure you have gathered together everything you need and are yourself ready to engage. Individuals with dementia may have a short attention span and will lose their focus if you are not ready when they are ready.

- *Simplicity*: Do not over-complicate arrangements or be too elaborate, because the emphasis will shift from the interaction to the arrangements around it. Some of the most successful interactions happen spontaneously.

Examples of positive interactions

A positive interaction often brings pleasure, but not all positive interactions have to be enjoyable. Some provoke deep emotions, including sadness, where a person may well cry or express anger. However, what makes the situation positive is how the individual concerned feels during and afterwards, having expressed emotion and been listened to.

Your assessment criteria:

DEM 312

4.2 Demonstrate a positive interaction with an individual who has dementia.

DEM 308

2.1 Give examples of positive interactions with individuals who have dementia.

2.2 Explain how positive interactions with individuals who have dementia can contribute to their wellbeing.

2.3 Explain the importance of involving individuals with dementia in a range of activities.

3.3 Describe how the environment might affect an individual with dementia.

? Reflect

Try to recall the three most positive and recent interactions you have had with people with dementia, who you work with. What made these interactions positive? How can you extend the potential for future positive encounters?

How positive interactions contribute to wellbeing

Your assessment criteria:

DEM 312

4.3 Demonstrate how to use aspects of the physical environment to enable positive interactions with individuals with dementia.

When a care practitioner engages with an individual through an enjoyable task, such as flower-arranging, this positive interaction contributes to wellbeing because it:

- stimulates interest

- provides activity and occupation

- maintains skills

- helps to build a relationship

- provides a sense of achievement.

Other general features of a positive interaction are set out in the Figure 2.12:

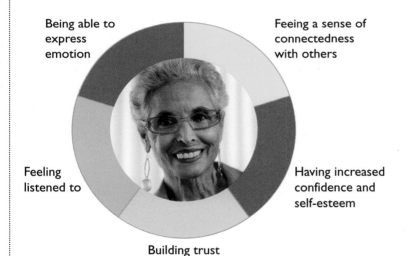

Being able to express emotion

Feeing a sense of connectedness with others

Feeling listened to

Having increased confidence and self-esteem

Building trust

Figure 2.12 Features of a positive interaction

Using the physical environment

The physical environment in which a person with dementia lives provides the context in which positive interactions take place. The environment is not just a building or outside space, but also the lighting, sound, furniture and layout. As a care practitioner you can use the environment, both inside and outside, to promote positive interactions.

The layout of a communal room should be conducive to one-to-one and group interaction, with the potential for a range of different seating plans to accommodate intimate conversation and larger groups.

 Discuss

Talk together with colleagues about ways to use the physical environment to good effect. For example, if you work in a care home, you could hold a DVD night and make the living room as much like a cinema as possible, for instance providing typical snacks such as popcorn and ice-creams.

A person's bedroom can contain familiar furniture from home that helps a person to feel safe, as well as prompting memories and reflecting the person's own identity. Bedroom furniture should be accessible to the person, for example not just a place for storage but a place where it is possible to view and select clothes and where positive interaction can take place to support decision-making about clothing suitable for the weather. Some care homes provide residents with a key to their room, which promotes a sense of personal ownership and privacy, allowing a person to invite you into his or her space, which is a positive interaction in itself.

Areas within a care setting, such as the dining room or sitting room, should be clearly designated to avoid confusion, and signs should show which rooms are which, so that residents know where to go at meal times and where to go when it is time to relax.

For those who like to be outside, any form of exercise is beneficial as it increases energy levels and stimulates the appetite. Opportunities for positive interaction are plentiful if people walk together around the garden, or just sit and enjoy the fresh air. Naming flowers, trees, shrubs and birds is an excellent way of practising recall, and demonstrating such knowledge can improve self-esteem. Every season brings different plants and flowers to look at, so this is an activity that can be repeated on a regular basis.

If a person is unable to go into a garden it is possible to bring the outside in through indoor plants and perhaps even a water feature, and bird feeders can be located near windows.

Finding suitable activities for each individual is important to provide stimulation, and taking part may provide opportunities for positive interactions.

Using the social environment

It is important to involve individuals with dementia in a range of social activities, because the nature of the condition means that without encouragement individuals increasingly withdraw into their own world, and opportunities for positive interaction diminish. Social opportunities can take place in groups, or some may be pursued as individual activities and may arise through:

- attending religious services

- going to clubs

- following sports

Discuss

Talk together with colleagues about the links the service you work within has with the wider community. Consider whether there are ways to increase and expand these.

Your assessment criteria:

DEM 312

 4.4 Demonstrate how to use aspects of the social environment to enable positive interactions with individuals with dementia.

- playing games, such as card or board games

- pursuing hobbies

- maintaining social routines, such as the services of a hairdresser or chiropodist

- eating out

- sharing memories and experiences.

Opportunities should be made available for the individual to meet with family and friends, who could be encouraged to take the person out or engage in a social event within the care setting.

Using reminiscence

Reminiscence techniques are part of a person-centred approach to care that places the individual at the heart of the activity. The person is encouraged to recall memories of past events using a variety of objects and stimuli as prompts. It is a useful form of interaction for people who have problems communicating verbally, because it uses the senses. It stimulates taste, touch, smell, vision and hearing in order to use the memory function, enabling the individual to draw on long-term memories as opposed to more recent ones. The techniques can be used on an individual basis, within a group at the setting, or by the family.

When a structured session is being organised, adequate time should be allowed for the recall of information as this does not happen instantly. Also, time is needed to relax after the session, which can be emotionally draining. Most libraries stock information on reminiscence techniques and can provide books and papers relating to such subjects as the Second World War, the 1940s, 1950s and 1960s, for example. Some museums can also lend memorabilia for reminiscence, such as pre-decimal coins, an old-fashioned iron and washing mangle and so on. Figure 2.13 on page 70 provides ideas for items to evoke reminiscence.

You can also ask questions to prompt reminiscence, although your emphasis should be on listening and not on asking too many questions. Some ideas are:

- Did you like school?

- What did you learn at school?

- What work did you do?

- What is your earliest memory?

Your assessment criteria:

DEM 312

4.5 Demonstrate how reminiscence techniques can be used to facilitate a positive interaction with the individual with dementia.

Key term

Reminiscence: *recollection of the past events of one's life*

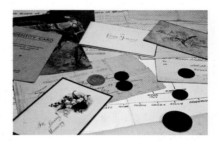

Reflect

Be aware that some individuals may not want to re-examine unhappy times from the past, and it might be necessary to avoid certain subjects, which friends and family should advise you about.

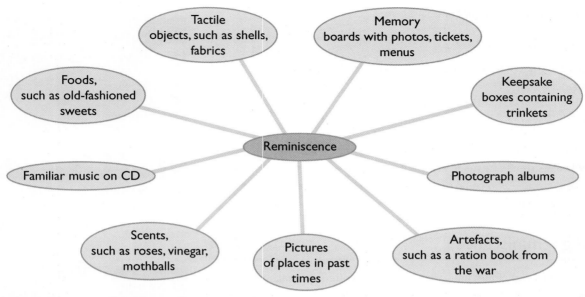

Figure 2.13 Examples of items for reminiscence

Case study

Angus used to live at home with his wife, but recent deterioration in his mental health because of Alzheimer's disease means he is undertaking a four-week trial in a care home. Angus once had a prestigious job as a civil servant and tells staff he likes things to be organised and in order. He has remained active since retirement, playing golf and enjoying many foreign holidays with his wife. They have four children and many grandchildren who visit when they can. Angus retains some insight into his condition and knows his memory is poor, constantly asking staff to remind him of the date and time. When family members visit he asks staff to prompt him about what he has been doing so he can tell them.

1. How might reminiscence techniques provide positive interactions with Angus?

2. How could you use the physical environment to engage Angus in positive interactions?

3. How could you use the social environment to engage Angus in positive interactions?

 Investigate

Using work, library and internet sources, find out about reminiscence services in your area. This might include a library or museum that lends artefacts and memorabilia, or a theatre or music group who put on shows specifically for older people. Why not make some enquiries and see what they can offer the service you work within.

Practical Assessment Task

This assessment task covers DEM 312 4.2, 4.3, 4.4, 4.5.

The ways in which you communicate and interact with individuals with dementia should be positive: they should be person-centred, supportive, enabling and recognise the unique identity of individuals. Positive interactions take place through activities that use the physical and social environments and reminiscence techniques. To complete this assessment activity you must demonstrate one or more positive interactions with an individual who has dementia which:

1. *use aspects of the physical environment*

2. *use aspects of the social environment*

3. *are facilitated through reminiscence techniques.*

Your evidence must be based on your practice in a real work environment and must be witnessed by or be in a format acceptable to your assessor. Keep any written work you produce, such as life-story work or care plans, as evidence.

Knowledge Assessment Task

This assessment task covers DEM 308 2.1, 2.2, 2.3, 3.3.

Positive interactions with individuals with dementia can take place through a range of activities and in different environments in ways that contribute to the person's wellbeing. To complete this activity you need to imagine you have been asked by your manager to make a presentation to your colleagues about achieving positive interactions with people with dementia through activities. Your presentation should include:

1. *an explanation of why it is important for individuals to be involved in a range of activities*

2. *a description of the ways in which these contribute to wellbeing*

3. *examples of four activities, two of which cater for individuals and two for groups of people with dementia, and which take into account the contribution of the physical environment.*

Keep the written work you produce for this activity as evidence towards your assessment. Your assessor may also want to ask you questions about the way you communicate with individuals with dementia in the work setting.

Assessment checklist

In order to successfully complete the unit, you will be required to produce evidence of your knowledge of dementia. The knowledge-related assessment criteria are show in the 'What you need to know' table below. You will also need to demonstrate your practical skills in communicating and interacting with individuals with dementia. The practice-related assessment criteria are shown in the 'What you need to do' table opposite. Your tutor or assessor will help you to prepare for your assessment; the tasks suggested in the chapter will help you to produce the evidence that you need.

Assessment criteria	What you need to know	Assessment task
DEM 312		
1.1	Explain how different forms of dementia may affect the way an individual communicates	Page 47
1.2	Explain how physical and mental health factors may need to be considered when communicating with an individual who has dementia	Page 47
1.3	Describe how to support different communication abilities and needs of an individual with dementia who has a sensory impairment	Page 47
1.4	Describe the impact the behaviours of carers and others may have on an individual with dementia	Page 53
2.3	Analyse ways of responding to the behaviour of an individual with dementia, taking account of the abilities and needs of the individual, carers and others	Page 53
4.1	Explain the difference between a reality-orientation approach to interactions and a validation approach	Page 61
DEM 308		
1.1	Explain how individuals with dementia may communicate through their behaviour	Page 53
1.2	Give examples of how carers and others may misinterpret communication	Page 53
1.3	Explain the importance of effective communication to an individual with dementia	Page 56
1.4	Describe how different forms of dementia may affect the way an individual communicates	Page 47
2.1	Give examples of positive interactions with individuals who have dementia	Page 71

Assessment criteria	What you need to know	Assessment task
DEM 308		
2.2	Explain how positive interactions with individuals who have dementia can contribute to their wellbeing	Page 71
2.3	Explain the importance of involving individuals with dementia in a range of activities	Page 71
2.4	Compare a reality-orientation approach to interactions with a validation approach	Page 61
3.1	List the physical and mental health needs that may need to be considered when communicating with an individual with dementia	Page 47
3.2	Describe how the sensory impairment of an individual with dementia may affect their communication skills	Page 47
3.3	Describe how the environment might affect an individual with dementia	Page 71
3.4	Describe how the behaviour of carers or others might affect an individual with dementia	Page 53
3.5	Explain how the use of language can hinder positive interactions and communication	Page 53

Assessment criteria	What you need to do	Assessment task
DEM 312		
2.1	Demonstrate how to use different communication techniques with an individual who has dementia	Page 61
2.2	Show how observation of behaviour is an effective tool in interpreting the needs of an individual with dementia	Page 61
3.1	Show how the communication style, abilities and needs of an individual with dementia can be used to develop their care plan	Page 65
3.2	Demonstrate how the individual's preferred method(s) of interacting can be used to reinforce their identity and uniqueness	Page 65
4.2	Demonstrate a positive interaction with an individual who has dementia	Page 71
4.3	Demonstrate how to use aspects of the physical environment to enable positive interactions with individuals with dementia	Page 71
4.4	Demonstrate how to use aspects of the social environment to enable positive interactions with individuals with dementia	Page 71
4.5	Demonstrate how reminiscence techniques can be used to facilitate a positive interaction with the individual with dementia	Page 71

3 | Equality, diversity and inclusion in dementia care

DEM 310
LO1 Understand the concept of diversity and its relevance to working with individuals who have dementia

- ▶ Explain what is meant by the terms diversity, anti-discriminatory practice and anti-oppressive practice

- ▶ Explain why it is important to recognise and respect an individual's heritage

- ▶ Describe why an individual with dementia may be subjected to discrimination and oppression

- ▶ Describe how discrimination and oppressive practice can be challenged

DEM 310
LO2 Understand that each individual's experience of dementia is unique

- ▶ Explain why it is important to identify an individual's specific and unique needs

- ▶ Compare the experience of dementia for an individual who has acquired it as an older person with the experience of an individual who has acquired it as a younger person

- ▶ Describe how the experience of an individual's dementia may impact on carers

- ▶ Describe how the experience of dementia may be different for individuals who have a learning disability, who are from different ethnic backgrounds, or who are at the end of life

DEM 310
LO3 Understand the importance of working in a person-centred way and how this links to inclusion

- ▶ Explain how current legislation and government policy supports person-centred working

- ▶ Explain how person-centred working can ensure that an individual's specific and unique needs are met

- ▶ Describe ways of helping an individual's carers or others understand the principles of person-centred care

- ▶ Identify practical ways of helping the individual with dementia maintain their identity

DEM 304
LO1 Understand key legislation and agreed ways of working that support the fulfilment of rights and choices of individuals with dementia while minimising risk of harm

▶ Explain the impact of key legislation that relates to fulfilment of rights and choices and the minimising of risk of harm for an individual with dementia

▶ Evaluate agreed ways of working that relate to rights and choices of an individual with dementia

▶ Explain how and when personal information may be shared with carers and others taking into account legislative frameworks and agreed ways of working

DEM 304
LO2 Be able to maximise the rights and choices of individuals with dementia

▶ Demonstrate that the best interests of an individual with dementia are considered when planning and delivering care and support

▶ Demonstrate how an individual with dementia can be enabled to exercise their rights and choices even when a decision has not been deemed to be in their best interests

▶ Explain why it is important not to assume that an individual with dementia cannot make their own decisions

▶ Describe how the ability of an individual with dementia to make decisions may fluctuate

DEM 304
LO3 Be able to involve carers and others in supporting individuals with dementia

▶ Demonstrate how carers and others can be involved in planning support that promotes the rights and choices of an individual with dementia and minimises risk of harm

▶ Describe how a conflict of interest can be addressed between the carer and an individual with dementia while balancing rights, choices and risks

▶ Describe how to ensure that an individual with dementia, carers and others feel able to complain without fear of retribution

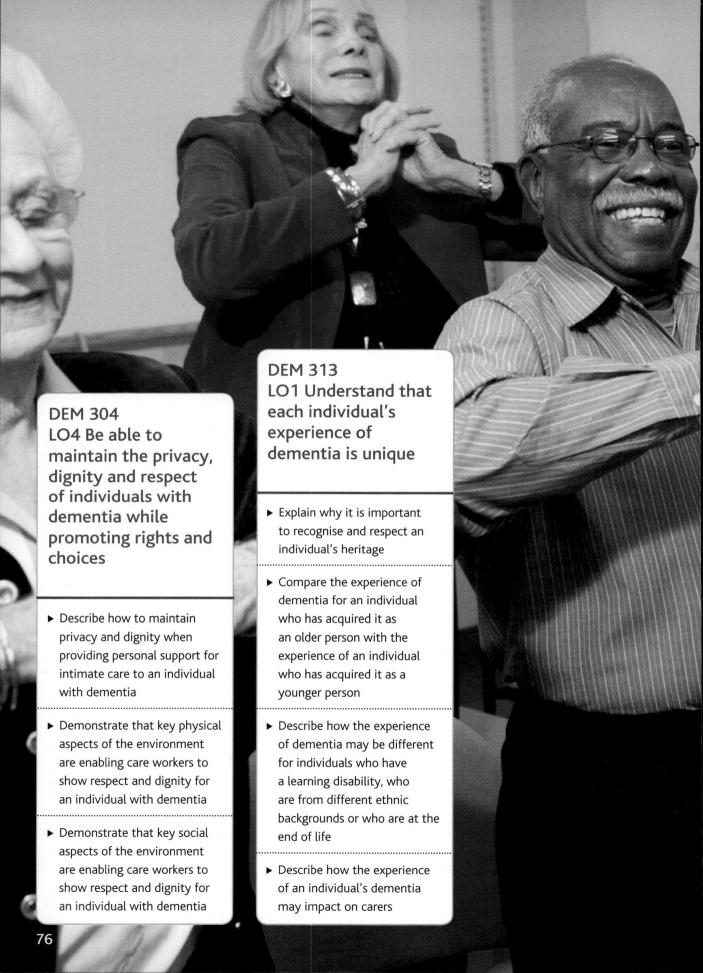

DEM 304
LO4 Be able to maintain the privacy, dignity and respect of individuals with dementia while promoting rights and choices

- ▸ Describe how to maintain privacy and dignity when providing personal support for intimate care to an individual with dementia

- ▸ Demonstrate that key physical aspects of the environment are enabling care workers to show respect and dignity for an individual with dementia

- ▸ Demonstrate that key social aspects of the environment are enabling care workers to show respect and dignity for an individual with dementia

DEM 313
LO1 Understand that each individual's experience of dementia is unique

- ▸ Explain why it is important to recognise and respect an individual's heritage

- ▸ Compare the experience of dementia for an individual who has acquired it as an older person with the experience of an individual who has acquired it as a younger person

- ▸ Describe how the experience of dementia may be different for individuals who have a learning disability, who are from different ethnic backgrounds or who are at the end of life

- ▸ Describe how the experience of an individual's dementia may impact on carers

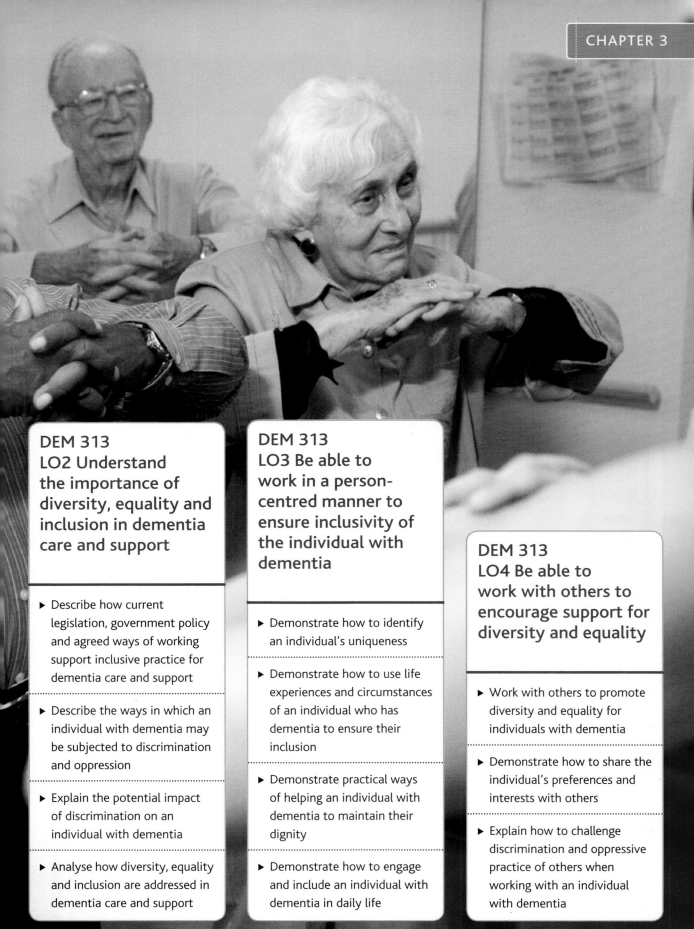

DEM 313
LO2 Understand the importance of diversity, equality and inclusion in dementia care and support

▶ Describe how current legislation, government policy and agreed ways of working support inclusive practice for dementia care and support

▶ Describe the ways in which an individual with dementia may be subjected to discrimination and oppression

▶ Explain the potential impact of discrimination on an individual with dementia

▶ Analyse how diversity, equality and inclusion are addressed in dementia care and support

DEM 313
LO3 Be able to work in a person-centred manner to ensure inclusivity of the individual with dementia

▶ Demonstrate how to identify an individual's uniqueness

▶ Demonstrate how to use life experiences and circumstances of an individual who has dementia to ensure their inclusion

▶ Demonstrate practical ways of helping an individual with dementia to maintain their dignity

▶ Demonstrate how to engage and include an individual with dementia in daily life

DEM 313
LO4 Be able to work with others to encourage support for diversity and equality

▶ Work with others to promote diversity and equality for individuals with dementia

▶ Demonstrate how to share the individual's preferences and interests with others

▶ Explain how to challenge discrimination and oppressive practice of others when working with an individual with dementia

Understanding equality, diversity and inclusion

Introduction to this chapter

This chapter focuses on the knowledge and skills you need to address a range of equality, diversity and inclusion issues that are part of dementia care practice. The chapter covers everything you need to know to complete three closely related units: DEM 310 *Understand the diversity of individuals with dementia and the importance of inclusion*, DEM 304 *Enable rights and choices of individuals with dementia while minimising risks*, and DEM 313 *Equality, diversity and inclusion in dementia care practice*.

Your assessment criteria:

DEM 310

1.1 Explain what is meant by the terms diversity, anti-discriminatory practice and anti-oppressive practice.

1.2 Explain why it is important to recognise and respect an individual's heritage (also **DEM 313 1.1**).

DEM 313

2.4 Analyse how diversity, equality and inclusion are addressed in dementia care and support

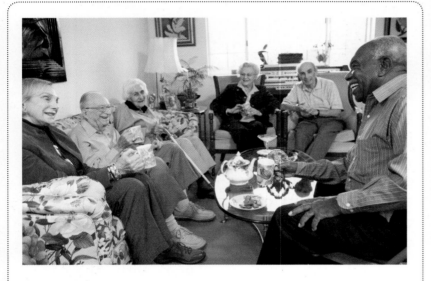

What are diversity, anti-discriminatory and anti-oppressive practice?

Diversity

As a health or social care worker you will work with colleagues, individuals with dementia, and other adults from a wide range of social, cultural, language and ethnic backgrounds. You will work with men and women, people with different types of ability and disability, individuals who speak different languages and who have different cultural traditions, as well as people who could be described as middle class, working class, as 'black', 'white' or of mixed heritage. The diversity of the people you work with and provide care and support for should be viewed in a positive way and as a reflection of wider society.

 Key terms

***Diversity**: difference or variety, the opposite of uniformity or sameness*

***Heritage**: biological, cultural and ethnic origins or background*

The diversity in the United Kingdom population is vast; if you think about the area where you live, you can probably identify a number of different local communities and groups. These differences impact on people's needs. As a result, you have a responsibility to understand and value difference as a way of meeting people's individual needs.

? | Reflect

Think about the individuals with dementia for whom you provide care and support. How diverse is this group of people? How do you acknowledge and respond to diversity in the way you practise at the moment?

Case study

Ena Goldberg, aged 90, is now unable to live independently. She has been diagnosed with dementia and has been supported at home by two care workers for the past two years. Like Ena, both of the care workers were Jewish and understood Ena's religious and cultural needs. Ena has very strong connections with the Jewish community and was a regular visitor to the local synagogue until recently. She is now too frail and unwell to attend. Ena's son is looking for a care home where staff will understand and be able to meet Ena's needs. He knows that Ena's faith and Jewish customs and traditions remain important to her.

1. How would you describe Ena's heritage?

2. What would you, as a health or social care worker, need to find out about to provide Ena with appropriate and respectful care and support?

3. Explain why Ena's cultural and religious background will have a significant effect on the care and support she requires.

Figure 3.1 Ethnic diversity in the UK (*Source*: Office for National Statistics)

Ethnic group	Population	Proportion of total UK population
White	54,153,898	92.1%
Mixed race	677,177	1.2%
Indian	1,053,144	1.8%
Pakistani	747,285	1.3%
Bangladeshi	283,063	0.5%
Other Asian (non-Chinese)	247,644	0.4%
Black Caribbean	565,876	1.0%
Black African	485,277	0.8%
Black (others)	97,585	0.2%
Chinese	247,403	0.4%
Others	230,615	0.4%

? | Reflect

Think about the different forms of diversity in your local area. Are there different ethnic communities, groups of people who speak languages other than English, or different religious communities, for example?

Investigate

How is diversity acknowledged and celebrated in the care setting where you work or where you are on placement? Find out about the way in which a person's background, abilities and achievements are assessed and documented, for example. You might also think about the ways in which care workers talk to the people they care for and support, and talk about them to others.

Understanding discrimination and its impact

Diversity is not welcomed or celebrated by everyone. Diversity and difference frighten some people, leading to a tendency to divide people into 'them' or 'us'. This can result in unfair treatment or discrimination against those who are different from the majority.

Unfair discrimination that is obvious and deliberate, and results in unfair treatment, is known as direct discrimination. For example, direct racial discrimination occurs if a care worker refuses to look after black residents, on grounds of their race or skin colour. Unfair discrimination that happens inadvertently, or is carried out in a secretive, hidden way, is known as indirect discrimination. Individuals with dementia can experience both of these forms of unfair discrimination.

Why do individuals with dementia sometimes experience discrimination and oppression?

There is some truth in regarding dementia as a destructive, incurable condition that is disabling and life-limiting. In the past this led to individuals with dementia being written off and devalued as people, as though their lives were over. The devaluing of people with dementia sometimes led health and social care workers to develop negative attitudes and impersonal approaches to care.

The discrimination and oppression that individuals with dementia sometimes experience tends to result from:

- **prejudiced** attitudes about dementia that stigmatise people with this condition and cause others to fear it

- the **stereotyping** and negative **labelling** of people who have dementia as 'dysfunctional', 'broken' and 'incapable' people

- the vulnerability of individuals with dementia, particularly where they are dependent on others for care, support or assistance

- the lack of a person-centred approach to meeting the care and support needs of individuals with dementia.

People who don't adopt a **person-centred** approach to dementia tend to regard individuals living with this condition as having become less than the person they once were. When this happens the person with dementia is diminished or even forgotten as an individual. This **dehumanising** approach to individuals with dementia strips people of their dignity, respect and human value, and increases the likelihood that their individual needs, wishes and preferences – and personhood – will be disregarded and devalued. Discrimination and oppression thrive in these

 Discuss

With a colleague or in a small group, try to identify a number of different ways in which individuals with dementia can be discriminated against. Consider whether the instances you identify are examples of direct or indirect discrimination.

 Key terms

Dehumanising: *making someone seem less human by taking away his or her individuality*

Labelling: *describing someone or something dismissively in a word (such as 'demented') or short phrase*

Person-centred: *focusing on an individual's particular needs*

Prejudiced: *based on a negative opinion, feeling or attitude; prejudices are typically based on inaccurate information or unreasonable judgments*

Stereotyping: *ill-informed, exaggerated and often prejudiced ways of thinking about a group of people*

circumstances because someone who is labelled as 'demented' isn't seen to have the same rights and human value as someone who is not.

How prejudice is expressed

Prejudice about dementia is expressed through the things people say and the way they behave towards individuals who have this condition. For example, prejudice:

- is often expressed through derogatory name-calling and by drawing attention to any physical frailty, mental health problems or cognitive difficulties (with memory or recall, for example)

- thrives where there is uncertainty, anxiety and fear about an individual or his or her dementia-based condition

- implies that people with dementia are less intelligent, less able or abnormal because of their condition

- treats individuals with dementia as inferior – less valuable, less worthy of attention and less deserving – because of their condition

- states that a person with dementia is wrong, 'broken' or dysfunctional, rather than just different.

? | Reflect

Think about the words and phrases that are associated with 'dementia care'. Make a list of the things that come to mind when you think about this. Are these words or phrases generally positive or negative? What do your family, friends and colleagues think 'dementia care' involves?

Case study

Anja is planning to open a small residential care home for people with early onset dementia. The residents will use the home for periods of respite care, staying for up to three weeks at a time. Anja has applied to the local council for planning permission to change the large house she now owns into care premises. Neighbours have been informed about the planning application and have begun a campaign against the project. They claim that the residents will be:

- unacceptably noisy and unpredictable

- unable to control their own behaviour

- frightening for local children and other residents

- at risk of getting lost or hurt by local traffic

- a nuisance to the local community.

The leader of the neighbourhood campaign group also believes that a dementia care home will cause the value of property to fall in the local area.

1. Identify the prejudices the neighbours have against people with dementia.

2. Describe how the neighbours of the proposed care home think about 'dementia' and the people who develop this condition.

3. Describe how you would feel if you were one of the prospective residents of the care home.

How discrimination affects people

Discrimination has a negative impact on individuals with dementia and may also impact on their family and friends. It is also negative for those who inflict discrimination – the perpetrators – because they fail to experience the benefits of diversity, equality and inclusion and the consequent broadening of their horizons.

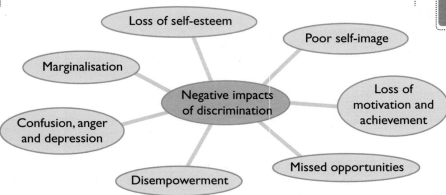

Figure 3.2 The negative impact of discrimination on individuals

Anti-discriminatory practice

Anti-discriminatory practice is an approach to care work that explicitly seeks to tackle unfair discrimination as a way of promoting the rights and equality of each person using care services. Unfair discrimination occurs when individuals or groups of people are treated differently, unequally and unfairly in comparison to others. For example, an employer who refused to interview candidates under the age of 25 for a dementia care job, saying 'in my experience, younger people are not good at relating to people with dementia', would be treating young people unfairly.

All users of care services should be treated fairly and equally. However, anti-discriminatory practice does not just mean treating everybody appropriately. It also means challenging and reducing any form of unfair discrimination that might be experienced by individuals with dementia.

 Discuss

Talk with colleagues or fellow learners about your experiences of discrimination.

- *Have you, or has someone you know, experienced discrimination?*

- *How did it make you (or the person you know) feel?*

- *What were the immediate and the long-term effects?*

Health and social care workers who take an anti-discriminatory approach are:

- aware of the different forms of unfair discrimination that can occur in dementia care settings

- sensitive to the ethnicity, social background and cultural needs of each individual for whom they provide care

- prepared to actively challenge and try to reduce the unfair discrimination experienced by people with dementia.

Anti-discriminatory practice is a way of **empowering** individuals with dementia to take control of their own care, support or treatment needs. It can be difficult to challenge instances of unfair discrimination or prejudiced attitudes. However, not doing so can mean that you get drawn in to reinforcing or supporting such discrimination. It is always better to draw your manager's attention to situations that you are concerned about or which you object to.

Anti-oppressive practice

Health and social care workers should always seek to meet the needs, wishes and preferences of individuals with dementia. The concept of working in partnership with individuals with dementia is now a very important part of person-centred dementia care. However, while the vast majority of people working in dementia care would see themselves as caring, some still work in a task-focused way and don't realise that they need to personalise the way they provide care for each individual. Where health or social care workers use their relatively powerful position to impose routines or perform tasks that an individual does not consent to, they are **oppressing** that person. This can happen in dementia care settings because individuals with dementia are often vulnerable and dependent on the people who provide care and support for them.

Health and social care workers who are aware of the power imbalance that is part of their care relationships can address this by working in an anti-oppressive way. For example, they avoid the use of care jargon or complex language that individuals with dementia cannot understand, and find ways of fully involving individuals in making choices and decisions about their own care and daily activities. These are examples of anti-oppressive practice. Health and social care workers who adopt an anti-oppressive approach find ways of working that maximise the involvement and control of the individual receiving care or support.

? | Reflect

Can you think of any instances where you have acted or worked in an anti-discriminatory way in a care setting? How could you adapt or develop your approach to care practice so that it became more anti-discriminatory?

✎ | Key terms

Anti-discriminatory practice: practice that challenges prejudice and unfair discrimination

Empowering: giving a person the power or authority to do or achieve something

Oppress: keep in a weak position through the use of force or power

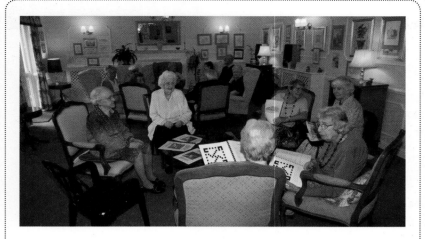

Challenging discrimination and oppressive practice

An anti-discriminatory and anti-oppressive approach to dementia care is based on ways of working that:

- recognise the individual needs of people with dementia from diverse backgrounds, including those who come from minority religious and cultural groups

- actively challenge the unfair discrimination and oppressive practices that people with dementia experience

- counteract the effects that unfair discrimination and oppression have already had on individuals with dementia.

Health and social care workers who want to challenge discrimination and oppressive practice should:

- be self-aware, self-critical and prepared to change their ideas and views about people with dementia

- continually develop themselves and reflect on equality and rights issues in the workplace

- be non-judgmental and regard people with dementia as being of equal value regardless of their physical, mental or cultural characteristics

- accept people's physical, social and cultural differences as a positive and interesting feature of dementia care work rather than something problematic

- become familiar with the equal opportunities policies and procedures of their workplace

- ask questions about, and seek advice on, ways of implementing the equality and anti-discriminatory policies and procedures of their workplace.

 Discuss

In a small group or with a colleague or your manager, identify and discuss examples of discriminatory or oppressive practice that you have seen or heard about. Why was practice discriminatory or oppressive in these situations? How were the situations resolved?

Difficulties of implementing anti-discriminatory practice

Promoting equality in the care setting means that health and social care workers need to address their own prejudices and tackle unfair discrimination where they see this occurring. This can be a daunting and intimidating task. Challenging incidents of unfair discrimination, or speaking out where people express prejudices about dementia, can require a lot of courage and personal confidence. Not everyone is able to do this. As a result, anti-discriminatory and anti-oppressive practice can be difficult to implement in settings where basic equalities issues have not been addressed and where there are weak procedures for complaints and whistle-blowing.

? Reflect

Have any of the care organisations where you have worked or undertaken work experience placements implemented an anti-discriminatory or anti-oppressive approach to care practice? If not, how do you think this would have improved practice?

Knowledge Assessment Task

This assessment task covers DEM 310 1.1, 1.2, 1.3, 1.4 and DEM 313 1.1, 2.2, 2.3, 2.4.

Health and social care workers should work in non-oppressive and anti-discriminatory ways when caring for and supporting individuals with dementia. A clear understanding of diversity, discrimination and oppression is needed to work in this way. With reference to dementia care practice in your workplace and the organisation where you work, produce a booklet or leaflet for new employees that:

1. *explains what you understand by the concepts of diversity, anti-discriminatory and anti-oppressive care practice*

2. *explains, using appropriate examples, why it is important to recognise and respect an individual's heritage when planning and providing care and support and communicating with them*

3. *describes how and why individuals with dementia may be subjected to discrimination and oppression*

4. *explains the potential impact of discrimination on an individual with dementia*

5. *describes how discrimination and oppressive practice can be challenged*

6. *analyses how diversity, equality and inclusion are addressed in the way dementia care and support are provided in your workplace.*

Keep your written work as evidence towards your assessment.

Diverse experiences of dementia

Diversity makes a difference

As a health or social care worker, you may already know that it is never a good idea to assume that because a group of people have one thing in common (such as their age, or a diagnosis of dementia) they will have other things in common too. This assumption is known as **stereotyping**. Stereotypical ideas about people with dementia can lead to care practices that are insensitive and inappropriate. Treating everybody as though they were the same – because they have 'dementia' – regardless of their individual needs, wishes, preferences and identity doesn't recognise individuality or acknowledge the importance of diversity. Understanding diversity is key to avoiding insensitive, outdated approaches to care practice.

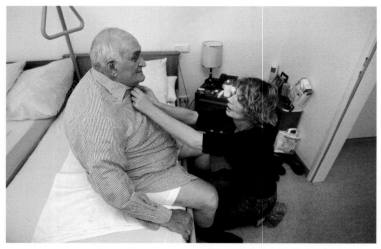

Diversity means the differences that exist between people. Differences relating to age, ethnicity and learning disability can make a difference to individuals' dementia care needs, their experiences of dementia and their preferences for how they want to receive care and support.

Younger people with dementia

Dementia-based illnesses are generally associated with older people over the age of 65. However, the Alzheimer's Society estimates that at least 16,000 people under the age of 65 are living with dementia in the United Kingdom today. This group of people often struggles to have their symptoms and problems recognised, and may be misdiagnosed as suffering from depression or stress, by medical practitioners who associate dementia with much older people.

Your assessment criteria:

DEM 310

2.2 Compare the experience of dementia for an individual who has acquired it as an older person with the experience of an individual who has acquired it as a younger person (also **DEM 313 1.2**).

2.3 Describe how the experience of an individual's dementia may impact on carers (also **DEM 313 1.4**).

Key term

Stereotyping: *ill-informed, exaggerated and often prejudiced ways of thinking about a group of people*

Investigate

Use an internet search engine to find out more about organisations that work with younger people who have dementia. Young Dementia and the Alzheimer's Society both have information on this area.

Despite the early age of onset, younger people who develop dementia-based conditions experience the same symptoms of memory loss, confusion and disorientation as older people. However, the care and support needs and problems that result from these symptoms may be different for younger people. For example, a younger person is more likely to have:

• significant financial commitments

• a job

• young or dependent children

• family responsibilities

• better general physical and mental health.

As a result, the services and facilities provided in a particular area for people with dementia may be unsuitable if they've been specifically planned and organised with older people in mind. Some dementia care services will also not admit or work with people unless they are 65 years old or more. This can lead to inadequate and inappropriate support for younger people with dementia and their families. While there is now more awareness of the needs of younger people with dementia and a growing number of services for them, provision is still variable and insufficient throughout the UK.

Investigate

What services or forms of support are available for younger people with dementia in your local area? Find out where people would be referred locally and what information, support or services are provided by your own care organisation (if any).

Case study

David grew up in the country. He graduated from university with a very good degree and went on to become an accountant. David was always good with numbers, very well organised and popular with his clients. David became a partner in an accountancy firm and was doing really well until about five years ago. When he was in his late forties things started to happen that worried his wife, Delia, and his work colleagues. David started to have trouble following simple instructions and began to make errors at work. At first colleagues covered up for him. David then began losing weight and behaving erratically. He would go out for a meeting and not return or would call to say he was lost. David was struggling so much that he was persuaded to take an 'extended holiday' from work. Delia did her best to support David and was extremely worried about him. When things reached the point where David just couldn't look after himself, he was admitted to a mental health unit for assessment. Not long afterwards, he was diagnosed with early onset dementia. He was 54 years of age.

1. How would you feel about working with a younger person with dementia, such as David?

2. How do David's support needs differ from those of an older person?

3. What, if anything, could be offered to David and his family by the care organisation where you work or by dementia care organisations in your area?

Knowledge Assessment Task

This assessment task cover DEM 310 2.2, 2.3 (also DEM 313 1.2, 1.4).

Health and social care workers who use a person-centred approach to practice understand that each individual's experience of dementia is unique. Recognising and understanding how an individual's stage of life and personal circumstances may impact on their experience of dementia is part of this. In this activity you are required to produce a case study that:

1. *compares the experience of dementia for an individual who has acquired it as an older person with the experience of an individual who has acquired it as a younger person*

2. *describes how the experience of an individual's dementia may impact on carers.*

Keep your written work as evidence towards your assessment.

Dementia and ethnicity

Individuals with dementia may belong to any ethnic group and may have a cultural or religious background that is important to their sense of identity. The Alzheimer's Society estimates that there are about 11,000 people from black and minority ethnic (BME) groups with dementia in the United Kingdom. Approximately 6% of this group are younger people with early onset dementia. Services for people with dementia from BME communities can be inappropriate and inaccessible where cultural identities, beliefs and traditions, as well as language differences, are not catered for. To avoid this, health and social care workers should find out about each individual's background and values and about the rules, beliefs, customs and traditions that are part of this. To practise in a respectful and sensitive way you will need to know how a person's cultural or religious values and background affect:

• what they can eat

• how they dress

• ways of undressing

• personal care issues

• what they feel about physical contact and being touched.

Dementia care services do tend to adapt to the needs of people from BME backgrounds where there is a significant local community of BME people. This is more likely to be the case in larger cities than in towns or villages. Outside of major cities, services for people with dementia from BME backgrounds may be not be seen as accessible or appropriate for meeting their particular needs.

Your assessment criteria:

DEM 310

2.4 Describe how the experience of dementia may be different for individuals who have a learning disability, who are from different ethnic backgrounds or who are at the end of life (also **DEM 313 1.3**).

? Reflect

How ethnically diverse is your local area? Does your care setting provide culturally appropriate care for members of the different ethnic groups in your local area? If not, how do you think this might be improved?

Learning disability and dementia

Learning disabilities can be caused by genetic disorders, such as Down's syndrome, by brain injuries or by pre- or post-natal infections, for example. A learning disability is not an illness, but it will affect a person's ability to cope with everyday activities throughout life.

People with learning disabilities are not typically associated with dementia. However, members of this group are at greater risk of developing dementia than non-learning disabled people.

Individuals who have Down's syndrome are at particular risk. Prasher's (1995) research indicates that the older a person with learning disabilities is, the greater the risk of developing dementia.

Prasher (1995) suggests that the following percentages of people with Down's syndrome have dementia:

- 30–39 years: 2%
- 40–49 years: 9.4%
- 50–59 years: 36.1%
- 60–69 years: 54.5%

Dementia affects learning-disabled people in much the same way as it affects non-learning-disabled people. However, the onset of dementia may be more difficult to detect and diagnose in learning-disabled individuals. This is linked to the reduced communication ability that learning-disabled people tend to have.

For example, individuals with learning disabilities may struggle to express how their abilities have deteriorated. They may not be able to explain their feelings of confusion, disorientation or difficulties with recall very clearly if they have limited verbal skills and vocabulary.

Close family members, carers or health and social care workers who are in close contact with the individual are likely to be first to notice the kind of changes in a person's behaviour or personality that are symptoms of dementia.

Key term

Learning disability: reduced intellectual ability and difficulty with everyday activities.

Investigate

Try to find out more about learning disabilities, particularly Down's syndrome, and how they affect people's everyday living skills. Information is available on websites and in a variety of textbooks on care and learning disability.

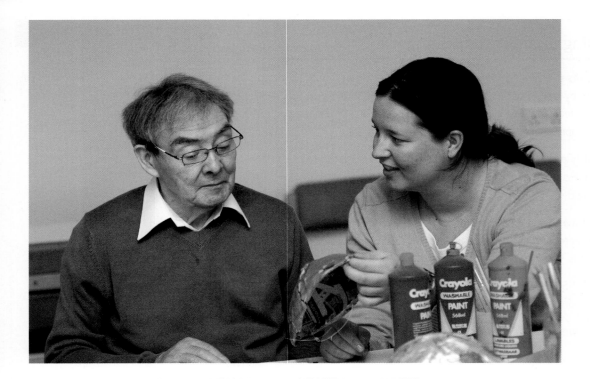

Supporting learning-disabled people

People with learning disabilities who develop dementia-based illnesses are best supported through a person-centred approach that focuses on their strengths, the skills and abilities they retain, and their interests. Health and social care workers should promote the independence and quality of life of learning-disabled people with dementia while minimising risk. In particular, it is important to:

- encourage the person to use both verbal and non-verbal ways of expressing thoughts and feelings

- give the person plenty of time and reassurance, listening actively and carefully to verbal and non-verbal communication

- support the person to manage the activities of daily life without taking over or doing too much in a way that is deskilling or undermining

- establish and reinforce clear activities of daily living routines to help the person to meet his or her own needs and feel confident about self-care

- use visual labels and images – as well as non-verbal communication – to help the person communicate and find the way around the home or care environment

- try to ensure that the person's living environment is quiet, calm and relaxed to prevent disturbance and minimise aggressive behaviour.

Case study

Elizabeth is 46 years old and has Down's syndrome. She lives independently in a supported housing flat and managed to look after herself, with occasional support from community workers, until a year ago.

Elizabeth fell in the bathroom of her flat while having a shower, breaking her wrist and bruising her ribs. Elizabeth's self-confidence declined markedly after this incident.

During a weekend stay at a specialist care home, staff noticed that Elizabeth was easily confused by what was going on around her. Following a full mental health and physical assessment, Elizabeth was diagnosed as having dementia, probably Alzheimer's disease. The psychiatric team diagnosing her felt that she had probably had the condition for some time.

1. What factors may have made it difficult to diagnose Elizabeth's dementia-based condition?

2. Which features of learning disability would care workers need to take into account when supporting or providing care for Elizabeth?

3. Should Elizabeth be supported to carry on living independently in her flat or do you think this is inadvisable?

? | Reflect

Have you ever provided care or support for an individual with learning disabilities? What kind of support or assistance did the person require? Were you also able to encourage and support the person to use the skills and abilities they did have to control aspects of their everyday life independently?

Dementia and end-of-life care

Individuals with dementia live for approximately 8, but sometimes up to 15, years following diagnosis. A person may die as a result of:

- complications arising from the end-stage dementia condition

- another illness (such as a cancer) during the earlier or middle stages of dementia

- a mixture of mental and physical health problems where dementia interacts with other conditions.

A person in the final stages of dementia is likely to experience a range of physical symptoms, including loss of appetite, low mood, pain and incontinence, as well as mental confusion. The physical and psychological care needs are considerable, and similar to those of people dying as a result of cancer.

Health and social care workers who provide care and support at the end of an individual's life should focus on:

- communicating as effectively as possible with the person to identify physical needs and reduce pain, discomfort and confusion as much as possible

Investigate

How are people in the final stages of dementia provided with care in your work setting? Find out what 'end-of-life' care involves where you work by asking senior colleagues or your manager.

- obtaining information from and working with palliative care specialists to provide effective and compassionate end-of-life care

- the quality and comfort of an individual's life, rather than on extending it through the use of invasive technologies such as artificial hydration and nutrition via tubes; one-to-one care and sips of water to moisten a person's mouth are more appropriate ways of alleviating pain, distress and discomfort in the final stages of dementia

- ensuring a person's religious or spiritual needs are recognised and met

- following a person's expressed wishes, including those expressed through an advanced decision (living will), verbally or in writing, at an earlier stage of a person's dementia

- involving carers and relatives of the individual with dementia in decisions about end-of-life care.

A person with dementia who is at the end of life requires good quality palliative care that ensures a minimum of discomfort and recognises rights, wishes and preferences. Health and social care workers play a vital role in providing compassionate care in these circumstances and must, to the very end of a person's life, recognise and respect his or her value as a human being.

Investigate

Using an Internet search engine, find the End of Life Care Strategy produced by the Department of Health in 2008. Identify the key points the strategy makes about the provision of care for people with dementia.

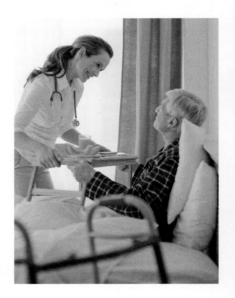

Knowledge Assessment Task

This assessment task covers DEM 310 2.4 (also DEM 313 1.3).

Individuals with dementia are a diverse group of people. One person's experience of dementia may be very different to another person's because of age, personal characteristics or cultural background, for example. In this activity you are asked to produce a summary table that describes how the experience of dementia may be different for individuals:

1. *who have a learning disability*

2. *who are from different ethnic backgrounds*

3. *who are at the end of life.*

Keep your written work as evidence towards your assessment.

Person-centred dementia care

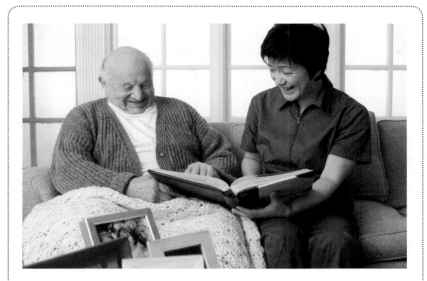

Your assessment criteria:

DEM 310

2.1 Explain why it is important to identify an individual's specific and unique needs.

DEM 313

3.1 Demonstrate how to identify an individual's uniqueness.

Specific and unique needs

Health and social care workers should always provide care and support that meets the specific and unique needs of each individual they work with. The **person-centred** approach to dementia care does this by:

- acknowledging and respecting the diversity of people with dementia

- ensuring that each person is treated equally and fairly

- including individuals in all aspects of care practice and daily life.

The person-centred approach to dementia care puts the person at the centre of the care planning, support and delivery process. It is based on the values of:

- individuality – recognising the uniqueness of the individual

- rights – ensuring individual rights are maintained

- choice – ensuring care or support is led by the individual's choices

- privacy – ensuring the individual is free from unwanted intrusion by others

- independence – enabling the individual to achieve maximum independence

- dignity – supporting the individual to maintain emotional control and a sense of worth in difficult and sensitive situations

 Key term

Person-centred care: *care that focuses on an individual's particular needs, wishes and preferences*

- respect – recognising and valuing the individual's sense of worth and importance to others

- partnership – working with others to achieving the best possible outcomes.

Using a person-centred approach is beneficial to individuals who have dementia because it focuses health and social care workers on improving each person's experience of everyday life, and extends their cognitive function.

Recognising individuals' unique needs and preferences

From a person-centred perspective, each person with dementia is a unique individual with a specific combination of physical, social and psychological qualities, characteristics, personality and heritage. An individual's personal background and life experience are also likely to have a direct impact on care and support needs, wishes and preferences. This is why it is important for health and social care workers to understand the *individual* with dementia as well as the illness.

To get to know the person as a unique individual, you need to:

- listen to what the person has to tell you

- talk to the person's partner and relatives

- obtain as much information about current abilities and skills as possible

- use all of this information to understand the person as an individual and to shape the way you work with him or her.

It is essential that health and social care workers get to know the person they are providing care for. Careful, active listening and observation of an individual will enable you to learn quite a lot over time. Even those people with limited ability to hold a conversation may be able to indicate non-verbally their likes and dislikes or the things that interest them. An individual's partner, relatives or close friends may also be able to provide you with valuable information about the person's history, past and current interests as well as particular likes and dislikes.

Case study

Brendan is an 84-year-old man with dementia. He is physically fit, but struggles to communicate verbally. Brendan is happiest when moving about. He constantly walks the corridors of the nursing home where he now lives.

Some of the other residents find this disturbing and shout at him to sit down. Brendan can become quite distressed when this happens, and can get very agitated (and even aggressive) if anyone tries to make him sit down. Brendan waits by the front door of the home and tries to slip out when it is opened. As a result he regularly goes missing. He is always found walking in the nearby park.

The new manager has asked Jo to become Brendan's key worker. Because little is known about his personal history, Jo arranged a meeting with Brendan, his wife and his son to find out more about him.

Jo discovered that before he retired, Brendan had been a postman for 20 years. He was also a keen cyclist and a prize-winning gardener. Roses were his special interest. Brendan's son also told Jo that he was researching their family tree, so Jo talked to him about putting together a life-story book that could be used to help Brendan remember and to encourage him to communicate. Brendan's family are keen to help with this.

1. How do you think Brendan's personal history may be influencing his current behaviour?

2. How could you use Brendan's interests and likes to plan his day-to-day activities?

3. How do you think a better understanding of Brendan's life history could enable care workers to improve the quality of his life?

? Reflect

How do you find out about the likes and dislikes, interests and life history of the individuals you support and care for?

Helping others to understand an individual's specific and unique needs

It is important that everyone caring for an individual with dementia focuses on the person's particular needs and preferences. This includes the person's relatives and friends as well as other professionals.

Those close to the individual with dementia or who work regularly with the person are likely to be pleased and reassured if you are asking questions or are seeking information about the person. This is an indication that you are trying to understand the person's particular needs and preferences.

Your assessment criteria:

DEM 310

3.3 Describe ways of helping an individual's carers or others understand the principles of person-centred care.

3.4 Identify practical ways of helping the individual with dementia maintain their identity.

DEM 313

3.3 Demonstrate practical ways of helping an individual with dementia to maintain their dignity.

You can use the information that you obtain and your understanding of the person to:

- inform and educate colleagues and others who have professional contact with the person about particular care needs, wishes and preferences

- share ideas, approaches and information with carers and others close to the person to enable them to provide care and support for the person at home, or to include them in care-giving in a residential or in-patient setting.

The relatives and friends of a carer need to understand the experiences that the individual is having, and should also be aware of the care needs and preferences of the individual with dementia. It is helpful to involve carers in as much of the care planning and delivery process as possible.

Many carers may already have acquired care-giving skills and abilities, and may have a deep knowledge of the individual with dementia. Establishing an effective relationship with a carer is an important way of sharing knowledge and understanding and of valuing his or her contribution to meeting the person's needs.

? | Reflect

Are there any individuals with dementia in your work setting about whom you know very little? Who could you ask to improve your understanding of the person by finding out about their background and specific needs?

Knowledge Assessment Task

This assessment task covers DEM 310 2.1, 3.2, 3.3, 3.4.

The person-centred approach is a key feature of modern dementia care practice. In this activity you are required to produce a leaflet that could be used as part of an induction pack for new employees in your work setting.

Your leaflet should:

1. *explain why it is important to identify an individual's specific and unique needs*

2. *explain how person-centred working can ensure that an individual's specific and unique needs are met*

3. *describe ways of helping an individual's carers or others understand the principles of person-centred care*

4. *identify practical ways health and social care workers can help an individual with dementia maintain their identity.*

Keep your written work as evidence towards your assessment.

Drawing on life history, culture and skills

Interacting with service users and their families in ways that clearly demonstrate respect is a very important part of inclusive practice in health and social care settings. Everybody who uses your care setting should be valued and respected for who they are, whatever their physical characteristics or their social or cultural background.

People feel respected when you:

- treat them as equals while recognising their individual needs, wishes and preferences

- acknowledge and recognise that their beliefs, culture and traditions are an important part of who they are

- use inclusive, non-discriminatory language that avoids stereotypes, prejudices and stigmatising terms

- are open-minded and prepared to discuss their needs, issues and concerns in a way that recognises the unique qualities of each person, as well as the characteristics they share with others

- show interest in their cultural and religious traditions and take part in an appropriate way in celebrating festivals and events that are significant for them and their community.

The use of life histories or biographies is a good way of getting to know the individual with dementia and of facilitating positive interactions. The aim of the life history is to build up a picture of a person's life.

You can do this by asking the person questions about past life experiences, or using familiar artefacts – for example photographs, pictures and favourite music – to stimulate a conversation. Friends, family members and partners can also provide information and artefacts to help you piece together the individual's history.

It may be best to obtain the information over a period of several weeks in order to gain a full picture of the person's life. The health or social care worker should try to learn about the individual's childhood, family life, school and job history, as well as views on life, and should be able to build a mental picture of the individual as a person with a rich life history.

Your assessment criteria:

DEM 313

3.4 Demonstrate how to engage and include an individual with dementia in daily life.

Key terms

Life history: an account of a person's life story that describes their personal background and experiences

Stigmatised: treated in a negative, derogatory way

Practical Assessment Task

This assessment task covers DEM 313 3.1, 3.2, 3.3, 3.4.

This activity requires you to demonstrate through your own care practice that you are able to work in a person-centred manner to ensure that individuals with dementia are included in daily life and activities. In particular you need to show that you can do the following.

1. *demonstrate how to identify an individual's uniqueness*

2. *demonstrate how to use the life experiences and circumstances of an individual who has dementia to ensure their inclusion*

3. *demonstrate practical ways of helping an individual with dementia to maintain their dignity*

4. *demonstrate how to engage and include an individual with dementia in daily life.*

Your evidence must be based on your practice in a real work environment and must be witnessed by or be in a format acceptable to your assessor.

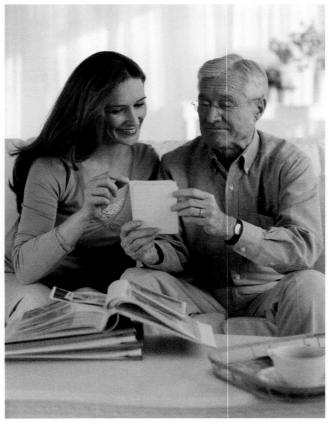

The use of life histories or biographies is a good way of getting to know the individual with dementia

Enabling rights and choices

The rights, choices and best interests of people with dementia should be a major concern for all health and social care workers. Legislation and the use of a person-centred approach are the two main ways of promoting inclusive practice for dementia care and support.

Legislation to enable rights and choices

Health and social care workers are required to work within a framework of laws, **policies** and **procedures** that set out standards for practice and agreed ways of working in dementia care settings. The purpose of key legislation is to protect and fulfil the rights and choices of individuals with dementia while minimising the risk of harm they may face in community or residential care settings.

The key points covered by a range of different laws are summarised in Figure 3.3 overleaf.

Your assessment criteria:

DEM 313

2.1 Describe how current legislation, government policy and agreed ways of working support inclusive practice for dementia care and support.

DEM 310

3.1 Explain how current legislation and government policy supports person-centred working.

DEM 304

1.1 Explain the impact of key legislation that relates to fulfilment of rights and choices and the minimising of risk of harm for an individual with dementia.

1.2 Evaluate agreed ways of working that relate to rights and choices of an individual with dementia.

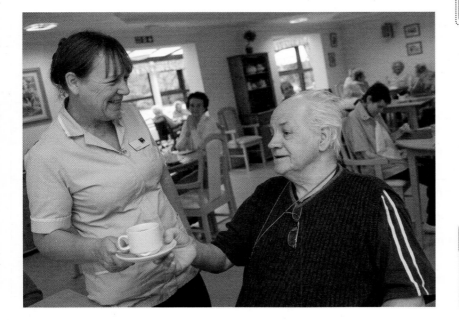

Key terms

Policy: plan of action

Procedure: way of doing something

Figure 3.3 Key legislation

Legislation	Key points
Human Rights Act 1998	Gives individuals a range of rights that must normally be respected by health and social care workers (see Figure 3.4 opposite)
	Individuals should be kept informed of their rights, including the right to access legal support if that is required
	Individual human rights can be overruled by care workers or relatives if the person poses a risk or is incapable of making a decision regarding his or her own welfare
Mental Capacity Act 2005	Every adult has the right to make his or her own decisions and is assumed to have the mental capacity to do so unless proved otherwise
	Individuals with dementia must be supported to make their own decisions and must be given all practicable help before it is concluded that they cannot make their own decisions
	People have the right to make eccentric or unwise decisions without being judged as lacking in capacity
	Decisions made on behalf of an individual without capacity must always be in his or her best interests
	Decisions made or actions taken on behalf of a person who lacks capacity should be the least restrictive intervention in terms of basic rights and freedoms
Adults with Incapacity (Scotland) Act 2000/2007	Assumes adults are able to make their own decisions regarding medical care unless proved incapable
	Judges an adult incapable if he or she is unable to make decisions, communicate decisions, understand decisions and retain a memory of them
	Allows adults to appoint a welfare attorney to make decisions for them in case their condition deteriorates to the point of being without capacity
	Provides that any intervention in the care of an incapacitated adult, either by a professional or welfare attorney or guardian, must benefit the individual, take account of his or her wishes and the views of others involved in care
Mental Health Act 2007	A person may be admitted to receive care or treatment against his or her will if mentally disordered
	Provides a right of appeal against compulsory admission and protection relating to treatment
Disability Discrimination Act 1995/2005	Prohibits discrimination against a disabled person, including individuals with dementia
	Places a duty on public authorities to promote equality of opportunity for disabled people
	Services must make 'reasonable adaptations' to enable disabled people to access and use services
Safeguarding Vulnerable Groups Act 2006	Restricts contact between vulnerable adults and those who might harm them
	Unsuitable people are barred from working with people with dementia
	Employers must check that a person is not barred from working with vulnerable people before employing him or her
	Assessment of suitability to work with vulnerable people should be on-going, not a one-off procedure

Legislation	Key points
Carers (Equal Opportunities) Act 2004	Gives carers who provide or intend to provide a substantial amount of care on regular basis the right to an assessment of their needs by a local authority
	Local authorities must take into account:
	– whether the carer works or wishes to work
	– whether the carer is undertaking or wishes to undertake education, training or leisure activities
	– support that can be provided from housing, health and education departments
	Gives carers the right to request flexible working hours from their employer
	Gives carers the right to information regarding the individual, provided that confidentiality is maintained

No Secrets (Adult Protection) is a UK government policy document that also provides guidance to local authorities on developing and implementing policies and procedures to protect vulnerable adults from abuse. The aim of the policy is to develop effective, multi-agency arrangements for safeguarding adults who are vulnerable to abuse. People with dementia should be covered by these arrangements.

Key terms

Confidentiality: privacy of information

Mental capacity: the ability to make decisions independently

Multi-agency: involving more than one care agency or organisation working together in a collaborative way

Safeguarding: protecting from danger and harm

Respect for private family life

Freedom of assembly and association

Life

Liberty and security

Freedom from torture and inhumane, degrading treatment

Freedom from slavery and forced labour

Fair trial

Human rights

Marriage and family

Freedom of expression

Freedom from discrimination

Freedom of thought, conscience and religion

No punishment unless in breach of the law

Figure 3.4 Rights protected by the Human Rights Act 1998

Health and social care workers need to understand how these laws provide a framework for their own care practice. There may also be circumstances where colleagues, carers or others require information and guidance on the rights of an individual with dementia.

Discuss

Which law protects the rights of the individual with dementia in each of the circumstances listed below?

- *a local café owner refuses to serve an individual with dementia because 'she's too messy'*

- *a person with dementia is given medication against his will when in hospital*

- *a relative wishes to take charge of the finances of a person with dementia*

- *a person with dementia is worried about being harmed by a care worker who visits her at home*

- *a residential home refuses to provide an adapted shower or bath for an individual with dementia*

Agreed ways of working

Health and social care organisations have a responsibility to ensure that their employees follow the laws safeguarding individuals with dementia in the way they provide dementia care and support. Care organisations do this by creating policies and procedures on agreed ways of working within their care settings. The policies and procedures should incorporate all of the legal requirements affecting care work.

It is therefore essential that health and social care workers understand and follow these policies and procedures. Failure to follow the agreed ways of working in a care setting may result in a health or social care worker ignoring safe systems of working, and not achieving the required standards or objectives of the care organisation. The worker could possibly be breaking the law and denying individuals with dementia their legal rights.

Investigate

Find out where the policies and procedures used in your workplace are kept and what they say about agreed ways of working in relation to health and safety, confidentiality and moving and handling situations.

Reflect

Why do you think it is important that every one of your colleagues understands and follows the agreed ways of working in relation to an area of practice such as moving and handling people or objects? What might be the consequences of not doing so?

Recognising mental capacity

Dementia-based illnesses are degenerative conditions. This means that individuals experience a gradual but inevitable loss of brain function. At some point, people with dementia-based conditions will lose their mental capacity. That is, they will become incapable of making informed judgments and decisions for themselves.

However, despite the likelihood of an individual with dementia losing mental capacity at some point, health and social care workers should not assume that a person with dementia is necessarily incapable of making decisions. Many people with dementia remain capable of making choices and of indicating their wishes and preferences until they reach the latter stages of their illness.

You should always try to offer individuals choice, support them in expressing their wishes, and respect their decisions. In order to achieve this it may be necessary at times to adapt the way you communicate with an individual and to be very sensitive to the way the person is able to communicate verbally and non-verbally.

Working in the least restrictive way

Many individuals with dementia are, or become, vulnerable and dependent. That is, they gradually lose the ability to manage their own safety and meet their own daily living and care needs. Health and social care workers who are aware of risk and the vulnerabilities of the people they work with need to find ways of working that avoid unduly restricting an individual's choices and freedoms.

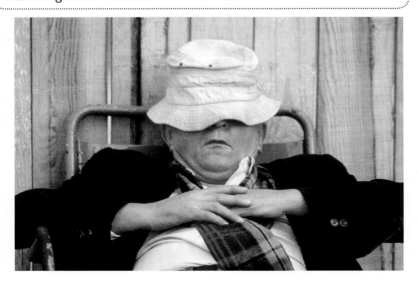

? | Reflect

Can you think of a situation in which you demonstrated respect for the mental capacity of an individual with dementia? Think about what you did and why you thought it was important to enable the person to make his or her own decision.

It is always important to manage risk, but at the same time individuals with dementia have the right to make their own choices and may behave in ways that seem eccentric, irrational or even embarrassing to others. In these circumstances, health and social care workers must respect an individual's rights and find the least restrictive way of providing the care, support and safeguarding the individual requires.

Discuss

With a colleague, or in a small group, discuss how each of the following workplace policies affects the way you work with individuals with dementia in your care setting:

- *moving and handling policy*
- *confidentiality policy*
- *equal opportunities policy*
- *safeguarding policy*
- *medication management policy.*

Case study

Farrah, aged 84, is a resident at Hinksey House, a residential and nursing care home. Farrah is one of the few residents who has a dementia-based condition. The staff at Hinksey House try hard to meet Farrah's needs but complain that there are too few of them, and that she needs constant monitoring.

Jean, a supervisor, is particularly concerned about Farrah's constant wandering. She believes that this is a health and safety risk, that it upsets other residents and takes up too much staff time to manage. Jean has started to block the entrance to Farrah's room with a safety gate normally used to stop babies and toddlers from wandering. Farrah can now see out and be seen by staff, but can no longer leave her room unaided.

1. Explain whether you think Jean's way of managing Farrah's behaviour is reasonable or discriminatory.

2. What impact might Jean's approach to this situation have on Farrah?

3. Describe what you think would be the least restrictive way of responding to Farrah's wandering behaviour.

Knowledge Assessment Task

This assessment task covers DEM 313 2.1 and DEM 304 1.1 and DEM 310 3.1.

Health and social care workers employed in dementia care settings must know about and work within a legal framework that protects the rights and interests of individuals with dementia and promotes person-centred working. In this activity you are asked to produce a booklet or poster that:

1. *describes how current legislation, government policy and agreed ways of working support inclusive practice for dementia care and support in your workplace*

2. *explains the impact of key legislation that relates to fulfilment of rights and choices and the minimising of risk of harm for an individual with dementia*

3. *explains how current legislation and government policy supports person-centred working in dementia care settings.*

You should keep a copy of the written work you produce for this activity as evidence towards your assessment.

Confidentiality issues

If you handle personal information relating to individuals with dementia, you are obliged by the Data Protection Act 1998 to protect that information. You should also be aware that an individual has the right of access to his or her personal information, according to a timescale determined by the Act. Though data protection law is very complex and continually developing, a key point to note is that health and social care workers must comply with the common law duty of confidentiality with regards to patient data.

An individual's consent must always be sought before information about him or her can be shared with others. Some good practice points relating to the sharing of information are as follows.

- Involvement of the carer in sharing information should not undermine the individual with dementia, who should retain a voice in decisions being made.

- An individual with dementia should be invited to any meetings the carer attends (rather than being excluded) so all parties are involved and are aware of what is taking place.

- If a health or social care worker is unable to share personal information about an individual with dementia with the carer(s) or others because the individual has not consented, the care worker should explain why as clearly and constructively as possible to minimise the development of mistrust or barriers to communication between the worker and the individual's carers.

- Policies on sharing confidential information with carers and others should be written and put into practice within the care setting.

- Clear boundaries need to be drawn regarding the sharing of information and an understanding of the individual's need for privacy.

- A person's care notes or records should document whether the individual has given consent to the sharing of specific information; consent should be informed, written, voluntary and recent.

It may be difficult for the health or social care worker to assess whether an individual with dementia has the mental capacity to make a decision about sharing information with carers and others. With earlier diagnosis and new treatments, people are retaining capacity for much longer, but in the case of those who are no longer capable, the Mental Capacity Act (2005) provides principles and guidance on this issue.

Your assessment criteria:

DEM 304

1.3 Explain how and when personal information may be shared with carers and others taking into account legislative frameworks and agreed ways of working.

? Reflect

Can you think of a time when a service user, member of their family or one of your colleagues confided in you and expected you to keep information confidential? Was this something you were comfortable with or did maintaining confidentiality make you feel under pressure?

Case study

Martin is admitted to your care setting for the second time, confused and in a state of neglect. He has been living on his own but is failing to cope. A neighbour, Sally, has been visiting him daily and providing him with cooked meals.

Martin refuses to allow staff to share any information about him or his health status with Sally, yet he wants to return home. It is clear, however, that Sally needs support in managing him so that he does not get into this neglected state again.

1. What rights and choices does Martin have?

2. What information could you share with Sally in this situation?

3. How could the Mental Capacity Act (2005) assist you in helping Martin to share his personal information with Sally?

Knowledge Assessment Task

This assessment task covers DEM 304 1.2, 1.3.

Health and social care practitioners should always be thinking about the effectiveness of the policies, procedures and agreed ways of working that influence their practice. This is a way of ensuring that individuals' interests are always at the centre of care practice.

In this activity you are asked to produce a short report that:

1. *identifies and describes two agreed ways of working in your work setting that relate to the rights and choices of individuals with dementia*

2. *evaluates each of the agreed ways of working by creating a table that lists the strengths and benefits of each way of working and the weaknesses or limitations of each way of working in relation to the rights and choices of individuals with dementia*

3. *explains how and when personal information about individuals with dementia may be shared with carers and others, taking into account legislative frameworks and agreed ways of working.*

You should keep a copy of the written work you produce for this activity as evidence towards your assessment.

The best interests of the individual

The best interests of an individual with dementia must always be considered when planning and delivering care and support. The Mental Capacity Act (2005) provides a list of factors that must be taken into account when deciding what is in a person's best interests. These include:

- the individual's past and present wishes and feelings, beliefs and values

- the possibility that the decision could be delayed if the person could regain capacity and the issue is not urgent

- the views of relatives and partners, as well as those of an attorney

- the need to avoid discrimination based on an individual's age, appearance, condition or behaviour

- the contents of any advanced statements

- the contents of any advanced directives.

The Mental Capacity Act (2005) states that every effort should be made to encourage an individual to take part in making a decision about his or her:

- finances

- health

- emotional and social wellbeing.

Your assessment criteria:

DEM 304

2.1 Demonstrate that the best interests of an individual with dementia are considered when planning and delivering care and support.

Key terms

Advanced directive: a 'living will' expressing preferences about medical care

Advanced statement: a statement about how future decision-making should be approached when the individual loses capacity

Discrimination: treating one particular group of people less favourably than another

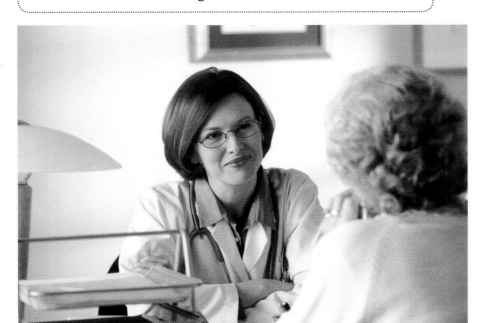

Discuss with a colleague in your practice setting how the best interests of individuals with dementia are being addressed. Talk about whether advanced directives are being used in practice, and how they could be used to maximise individuals' rights and choices.

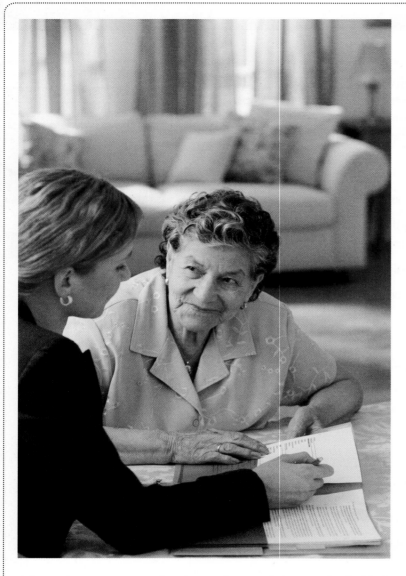

Advanced statements are clear instructions made by an individual before he or she loses capacity. Advanced directives deal specifically with the individual's wishes regarding future medical care, such as any refusal of treatment when the condition deteriorates. In order to make an advanced directive, the individual must be:

• competent at the time of the declaration

• informed about the procedure and what it will involve

• free from any undue influence.

Enabling rights and choices

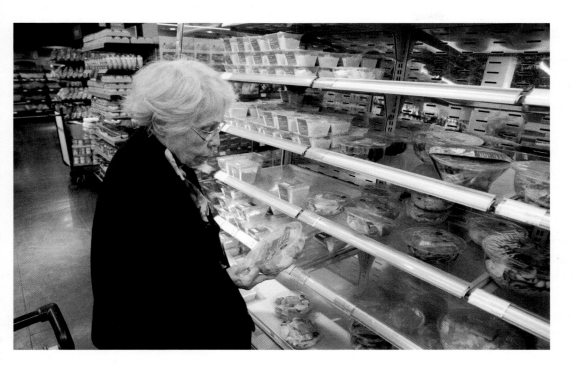

Supporting individuals to exercise rights and choices

It is important to recognise that individuals should be given the opportunity to exercise their rights and choices, even when their decisions are not necessarily in their best interests. Some negotiation may have to take place and a compromise may need to be reached if the desired choice could put the individual at risk of harm. When this occurs, the level of risk posed by a decision should be considered; risk is evident in all aspects of everyday life, and a certain level of risk may be acceptable. The Department of Health's *Ten Essential Shared Capabilities* (DH 2004) states that there is a tension between promoting safety and positive risk-taking. Essentially, the care team must be aware of risks, taking appropriate action when required, thus avoiding negligent practices.

Assessment of risk should be based on a multi-professional approach that also involves the individual with dementia. When conducting a risk assessment, the following should be considered systematically:

- any history of previous risky behaviours – ask the individual directly and research other information, including letters written regarding previous behaviour; involve carers and partners

Your assessment criteria:

DEM 304

2.2 Demonstrate how an individual with dementia can be enabled to exercise their rights and choices even when a decision has not been deemed to be in their best interests.

🔑 Key term

Compromise: *establishing a mutually agreed objective where each side has to make concessions until agreement is finally reached*

- patterns of any risky behaviour – are any behaviours repeated?

- recent risky behaviour – are there any recent incidents relating to the identified risk?

- documentation of risk – how is the risk being documented; is a policy in place?

- communication of risk – who needs to be informed?

Risk assessments are carried out on a regular basis to monitor, for example, clinical and environmental risks in the workplace setting. You need to identify where the records of risk assessments are located within your workplace setting, who has responsibility for conducting the risk assessments and auditing them, how often they are conducted and who carries out the relevant actions. The assessments should be made available to all health and social care workers and should not be a paper exercise – findings should be acted upon. In small settings, the audit may be carried out by the manager of the care setting.

Supporting decision-making

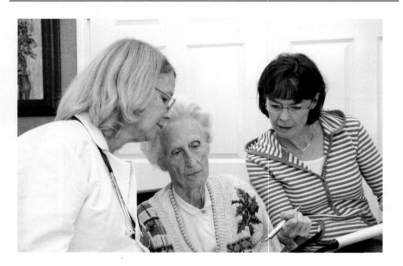

Do not assume individuals cannot make their own decisions

It should not be assumed that an individual with dementia cannot make decisions. Everyone has the capacity to make decisions until proven otherwise. A person-centred approach encourages a positive attitude to decision-making; the focus is on the individual's abilities and strengths rather than on the long-term condition. Person-centred care will consider the whole person, including whether that individual

Your assessment criteria:

DEM 304

2.3 Explain why it is important not to assume that an individual with dementia cannot make their own decisions.

2.4 Describe how the ability of an individual with dementia to make decisions may fluctuate.

still has the ability to make decisions regarding care. When the individual can no longer make decisions, his or her mental capacity is assessed by the caring team. The Mental Capacity Act (2005) provides principles and guidance to assist assessment.

The Act suggests that individuals should be given all necessary help to make supported decisions before it can be concluded that they can no longer make their own decisions. There is a two-stage test of mental capacity:

- Does the person have brain impairment, or is there something affecting how the brain works? Dementia is considered to be relevant here.

- If so, is the person unable to make a decision regarding the question that is being asked?

The Mental Capacity Act (2005) supports a 'functional' or 'decision' test that recognises that an individual's ability to make decisions could vary from time to time, depending on the stage of dementia and the type of decision that is being requested.

Some decisions are more difficult to make than others; for example, deciding what to wear is easier than managing one's financial affairs or deciding to sell one's home. So individuals may be able to make some decisions, but a failing memory may prevent them from making others.

An advanced directive is also known as a 'living will'. This enables individuals to make very important decisions regarding their future medical care. If these decisions are not made when individuals have the capacity, decisions could be made by others that go against their wishes.

Fluctuating decision-making ability

An individual with dementia may be able to make decisions in more lucid moments, even if these are fleeting. This may depend on the type of dementia and the stage of the disease. Those who have Alzheimer's disease do experience these moments, but these can be upsetting times if the individual realises that mental capacity is declining.

Even if individuals have memory loss and generally recall only past events, they may suddenly become fully aware of their present circumstances and may feel able to make important decisions; you should encourage them to be cautious. Carers should be aware of individuals' beliefs and values as these may influence decisions they wish to make.

During periods of awareness, the individual could be asked to consider advanced directives to plan for his or her future medical care. This will depend on how often the individual has these periods of heightened awareness, and whether he or she feels able to make such vital decisions.

? Reflect

Reflect on how you, as a care worker using the patient-centred approach, could help an individual to make a decision affecting his or her life.

- Refer to examples you have observed in your practice placement.
- Suggest how the Mental Capacity Act can assist you in helping the individual to make decisions.
- Discuss with your tutor and make notes in your journal.

Key terms

Risk assessment: a process that aims to identify potential risks to the health, safety and security of all people at a specified location

Lucid: clear, rational and aware

Case study

Stephen is an 80-year-old man who lives with his wife, Jean. Stephen lived an active life until about six months ago, when Jean noticed a change in his behaviour. He no longer went fishing, was neglecting his personal hygiene and was becoming increasing forgetful.

As Stephen has become increasingly difficult to manage at home, Jean has asked for respite care. However, Stephen has refused to be admitted.

1. What risks does Stephen pose by being at home in his current state?

2. How could you support Jean using the person-centred approach?

3. How can the Mental Capacity Act and advanced directives help Stephen in making decisions regarding his future care?

Practical Assessment Task

This assessment task covers DEM 304 2.1, 2.2, 2.3, 2.4.

Maximising the rights and choices of individuals is an important element of good practice in dementia care. You should focus your work for this activity on your own practice in relation to providing care for an individual with dementia.

You will need to do the following:

1. *demonstrate that the best interests of an individual with dementia are considered when planning and delivering care and support*

2. *demonstrate how an individual with dementia can be enabled to exercise their rights and choices even when a decision has not been deemed to be in their best interests*

3. *explain why it is important not to assume that an individual with dementia cannot make their own decisions*

4. *describe how the ability of an individual with dementia to make decisions may fluctuate.*

Your evidence must be based on your practice in a real work environment and must be witnessed by or be in a format acceptable to your assessor.

Maintaining privacy, dignity and respect through care practice

Providing intimate care

Health and social care workers should be able to meet the personal care needs and preferences of individuals with dementia in a supportive and dignified way. This might include assisting a person to:

- use toilet facilities
- bathe, wash or manage mouth care
- dress, undress or manage personal appearance.

Maintaining privacy when providing intimate care is always an important issue because:

- it affects an individual's dignity and self-respect
- the individual may be vulnerable
- the individual might feel he or she is a burden.

Health and social care workers need to:

- understand how individuals might feel in this kind of situation
- show respect for and sensitivity towards the person
- protect the individual's dignity when providing care.

How can privacy be maintained?

Individuals should always have privacy when personal care is being provided. When washing, dressing, bathing, or attending to other personal care needs, they should always be out of sight and – if possible – out of earshot of other people.

How you achieve this should be agreed with the individual and should follow the agreed ways of working for your work setting. Key points include:

- keeping the bathroom or toilet door closed and/or locked
- pulling curtains or a screen around the person's bed
- never leaving the individual partially dressed in view of others
- always knocking before you enter a private area
- talking quietly during care procedures so others can't overhear you.

Your assessment criteria:

DEM 304

4.1 Describe how to maintain privacy and dignity when providing personal support for intimate care to an individual with dementia.

4.2 Demonstrate that key physical aspects of the environment are enabling care workers to show respect and dignity for an individual with dementia.

4.3 Demonstrate that key social aspects of the environment are enabling care workers to show respect and dignity for an individual with dementia.

? Reflect

Think of the last time you provided intimate care for an individual at work. What did you do to protect dignity and to show respect?

? Reflect

Reflect on a time when you were involved in a sensitive personal care situation. How did you feel about either providing or receiving support?

Case study

Sheila has been diagnosed with the early stages of dementia and has recently suffered a stroke. She has lost the ability to speak as a result of her stroke and spends much of the day in a chair. When she wants something she uses flashcards. The set of flashcards helps her communicate when she is hungry, wants to brush her hair, or for any other issues that are important to her wellbeing and comfort. Stanislas, a care worker, is aware that the flashcards are used by Sheila when she wants to use the toilet. During the morning Stanislas notices that Sheila is looking at him. He goes over to her and suggests she uses the flashcards to say if she wants something. At first Sheila looks embarrassed, but then shows Stanislas the card with a picture of a toilet on it. Stanislas is about to help take Sheila to the toilet, when he remembers something else. He shows her the card with a picture of a woman on it. Sheila smiles and nods her head. Stanislas then goes to ask his colleague Maria to help Sheila. When using the toilet Maria leaves Sheila alone and knocks on the door after a few minutes to see if she is finished before helping her back to her chair.

1. Why might Sheila be reluctant to tell Stanislas about her personal care needs?

2. How does Stanislas encourage Sheila to communicate her care needs?

3. How does Maria help maintain Sheila's privacy?

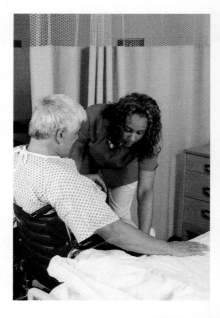

 Investigate

Investigate how individuals in your work setting are supported with their personal care.

Respecting personal, social and emotional space

Individuals with dementia may live in their own homes in the community or in residential settings such as nursing and care homes. The place a person lives in is usually personalised with pictures, ornaments and items of furniture that have special meaning for the person. An individual's personal environment, whether it is his or her own home or a room in a care home, may also give the person a sense of security and feel like somewhere the person can truly be himself or herself. Health and social care workers should always respect an individual's need to have such a personal space. The policies and procedures of care settings usually state that care workers should knock and gain permission before entering a person's room, and be respectful when working in a person's own home.

Giving individuals social and emotional space involves respecting their right to make choices about their social activity and their emotional involvement with others. Having opportunities to participate in everyday activities, and to make a positive contribution to community and society, helps individuals with dementia to avoid social isolation. At the same time, health and social care workers need to respect the right people have to choose whether or not, and with whom, they wish to socialise or form relationships.

Individuals with dementia may enjoy social contact and activities with others, but should always be given the opportunity to opt out or choose their own company too. It is important to ensure that vulnerable people, such as those with dementia, do not become socially isolated and are not put at risk because of privacy policies and that they are not emotionally manipulated or overwhelmed by the way others behave and relate towards them.

Valuing people in practice

An individual with dementia should always feel valued as a person. This means valuing people as they are today – not just valuing who they used to be earlier in life. Health and social care workers can help people with dementia to feel valued by:

- being flexible and tolerant in their approach to providing care and support

- including individuals in conversations about or relating to them, never talking over them or as though they are not present

- acknowledging that an individual is trying to communicate even when what he or she says is difficult or even impossible to follow

- giving people time to express themselves and to complete tasks, never criticising or telling them off for what they have or haven't been able to do

- providing the minimum level of support or assistance individuals require so that they can maintain their daily living skills and feel empowered and capable of doing as much for themselves as they are able

- being positive when communicating, and affectionate in ways that each individual feels comfortable with

- providing opportunities to be active and involving people in the kinds of activities they can actively take part in

- using each person's preferred title, name or nickname when communicating

- being kind and reassuring and never being off-hand, impatient or discourteous

- listening and trying to understand people's feelings, never brushing off their concerns or worries or dismissing them with comments such as 'cheer up' or 'never mind'.

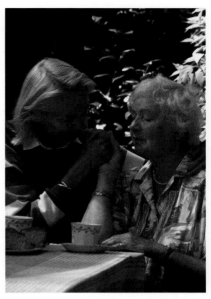

How do you value the people you provide care for?

> **? Reflect**
>
> *Think about how you value the people you provide care for through the way that you practise dementia care. How do you do this? Have you seen other colleagues do or say things that valued the people they were caring for?*

By valuing people with dementia you are recognising and respecting them as unique individuals. As well as focusing on who a person is, this approach acknowledges what people can still do, seeks to include them in their own care and engages them in daily life. You should:

- try to identify tasks or activities people can succeed at and avoid putting them in situations they can't cope with

- support individuals to complete tasks or activities at their own pace and in the way they prefer

- promote individuals' independence by doing things *with* them rather than *for* them

- promote individuals' sense of achievement and self-worth by enabling them to complete part of a task if they cannot manage it all.

? Reflect

How inclusive are you as a care practitioner? Do you encourage individuals to play a part in their own care, and encourage or enable them to participate in activities? If not, or if you would like to do this a little more, reflect on how others practise in a more inclusive way.

Practical Assessment Task

This assessment task covers DEM 304 4.1, 4.2, 4.3.

Individuals with dementia gradually lose their self-care skills, independence and ability to make decisions. As a result it is very important that health and social care workers act to maintain the privacy, dignity and respect of people who are no longer able to do this for themselves. In this assessment activity you need to show that you act to safeguard and maintain the privacy, dignity and respect of the individuals with whom you work. In relation to your own practice, you should complete the following tasks:

1. *describe how you maintain privacy and dignity when providing personal support for intimate care to an individual with dementia*

2. *demonstrate that key physical aspects of the environment are enabling care workers to show respect and dignity for an individual with dementia*

3. *demonstrate that key social aspects of the environment are enabling care workers to show respect and dignity for an individual with dementia.*

Your evidence for this task must be based on your practice in a real work environment and must be witnessed by or be in a format acceptable to your assessor.

Working with carers and others

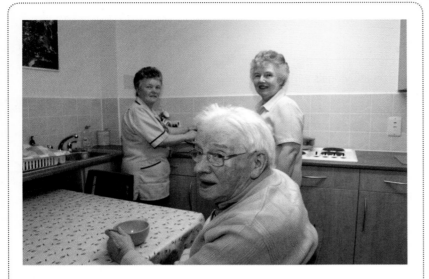

Your assessment criteria:

DEM 304

3.1 Demonstrate how carers and others can be involved in planning support that promotes the rights and choices of an individual with dementia and minimises risk of harm.

Involving carers in planning support

Carers commonly worry about individuals with dementia, including about what could happen if they leave the person unattended and how to cope with challenging behaviours. Carers have to cope with changing demands and unpredictable outcomes. Therefore, they require a lot of support and sensitivity.

As discussed in this chapter, the individual's best interests and preferences must take priority and be placed at the centre of all provision. This can be difficult for carers, who may feel that their own needs are neglected. Care planning should involve carers along with members of the multi-disciplinary team, and the plan should:

- promote the rights and choices of the individual

- minimise risk and harm

- provide equitable and individualised care, treating each person as an individual

- adhere to equal opportunities legislation and good practice

- recognise and value diversity

- promote anti-discriminatory practice

- adhere to the Human Rights Act (DCA 1998) – individuals should be informed of their rights.

Carers should be made aware of the confidential nature of the individual's personal information through involvement in care planning.

Conflicts of interest

Although carers should always try to impress on individuals with dementia that they have rights and choices, they will be aware of their dependence and can feel very vulnerable as a result. Nonetheless, most individuals want to retain some control over their lives, especially with regard to making decisions.

Carers may face a dilemma when they believe that they know what is best for a person, but the individual has conflicting ideas. However, carers should accept that the individual needs to retain some independence by taking control of some aspects of life, even though he or she may be vulnerable to risk.

Individuals with dementia and their carers are entitled to:

- opportunities to enhance their abilities

- participation in decisions that will affect their daily lives, now and in the future

- opportunities to participate in the wider community

- assessment of their general, medical and social needs.

How to enable complaints without fear of retribution

Every organisation should have a complaints procedure; an individual with dementia, carers and others should feel able to complain without retribution. A number of national organisations have complaints procedures, for example local authority social services departments, the NHS and the Care Quality Commission (DH 2009), the independent regulator of health and adult social care in England. The NHS Constitution (DH 2010) explains patients' rights when making general complaints about services within the NHS system. These include the right to:

- have a complaint dealt with efficiently and properly investigated

- know the outcome of any investigation into a complaint

- take the complaint to the Independent Parliamentary and Health Services Ombudsman if the patient is not satisfied with the way the NHS has dealt with it

Your assessment criteria:

DEM 304

3.2 Describe how a conflict of interest can be addressed between the carer and an individual with dementia while balancing rights, choices and risks.

3.3 Describe how to ensure an individual with dementia, carers and others feel able to complain without fear of retribution.

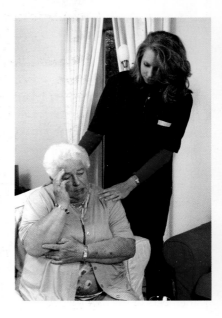

? | Reflect

Reflect on any dilemmas that you have observed while on your placement between an individual and his or her carer. How were these managed within the care setting?

- make a claim for a judicial review if the patient has been affected by an act or by a decision

- receive compensation following any harm.

? Reflect

What would you do if a service user or a relative told you that they wanted to make a complaint about an aspect of care practice in your work setting? Do you know enough about the complaints procedure to tell them how they can do this?

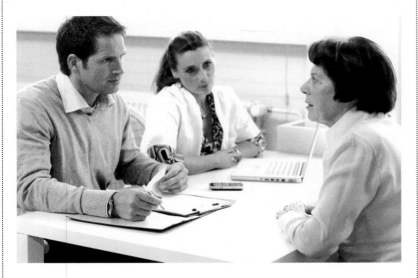

It is important that any complaint is made as soon as possible, and within 12 months of the event happening. Complaints can be made directly to the service in question or to the local Primary Care Trust that commissioned the care.

Since April 2009, each hospital or trust runs a simple complaints process. Patient Advice and Liaison Services (PALS) provides advice, helping relatives and carers on a wide range of issues that can be resolved quickly and easily. PALS usually encourages complainants to raise concerns with the member of staff concerned with the care.

Other services that can be accessed for support and guidance when making a complaint are:

- the Independent Complaints Advocacy Service, a national service

- the Citizens Advice Bureau, which provides support for complaints about the NHS, social services and local authorities.

Case study

Rita is 76 years old and lives at home with her husband, Angus, who has vascular dementia. If possible, she wants to continue caring for him at home.

Although they both attend a local support group once a week, Rita recognises that they both need more support, especially as Angus's mental capacity is deteriorating. He is becoming more confused. He has been admitted to a care home for assessment.

1. How would you support Rita in planning care for Angus, ensuring that he still exercises his rights and choices?

2. How would you manage the dilemmas of their conflicting interests regarding what he feels he needs and what she thinks he needs?

3. What advice would you give Rita if she decides to complain about his care?

Investigate

Using online and library sources, investigate the NHS and local authority complaints procedures that carers, others and individuals with dementia can access for information. Find out how your practice placement handles complaints.

Practical Assessment Task

This assessment task covers DEM 304 3.1, 3.2, 3.3.

Effective, person-centred care for individuals with dementia requires everyone involved with an individual to participate in the planning and delivery of care. Involving carers and others in supporting an individual with dementia requires a range of skills and abilities. In this practical activity, you need to show that you have these abilities.

Focusing on your own care practice, you should choose an individual with dementia with whom you work and do the following.

1. *Demonstrate how carers and others can be involved in planning support that promotes the rights and choices of the individual while minimising risk of harm.*

2. *Describe how a conflict of interest can be addressed between the carer and an individual with dementia while balancing rights, choices and risks.*

3. *Describe how to ensure an individual with dementia, carers and others feel able to complain without fear of retribution.*

Your evidence for this task must be based on your practice in a real work environment and must be witnessed by or be in a format acceptable to your assessor.

Involvement of carers

Every member of a family is likely to be affected by an individual's dementia. The way family members respond to a person with dementia is likely to depend on the quality of the relationships they had with the person before he or she developed the condition. Many relatives, particularly the partners of individuals with dementia, commit themselves to providing as much care and support for the person as they are able. This can become stressful, and it changes the lifestyle of the carer considerably. Health and social care workers can provide support and assistance for carers in a number of ways, including:

- listening to the concerns of carers in a genuine and supportive way
- discussing and suggesting safety measures to safeguard both the individual with dementia and the carer
- involving the carer in discussions about the individual's care with other key personnel (doctors, social workers, nurses)
- providing information and guidance on care-related issues through factsheets
- encouraging the carer to promote the independence of the individual and to maintain his or her own interests and activities outside of caring
- involving the carer in planning support and care for the individual
- discussing and identifying risks to the carer's own and the individual's health and safety
- encouraging the carer to make use of advocates and interpreters where these are required to get the best from care services on behalf of the individual.

It is always best not to advise the relatives of a person with dementia how they should live their lives or what they should do in particular circumstances. A partnership approach in which you provide support and suggestions is more helpful than telling people who are under pressure what they should do. Taking notice of what family members tell you about the individual and the care situation they face, and trying to understand their point of view, is a useful way of involving carers and likely to be reassuring to them.

Supporting carers

The carers of individuals with dementia are often very involved in providing care and support. It is important to recognise that this is a stressful role and that carers may themselves require care and support to cope with the demands made on them. Health and social care workers can make life easier and less stressful for carers by:

Your assessment criteria:

DEM 313

4.1 Work with others to promote diversity and equality for individuals with dementia.

4.2 Demonstrate how to share the individual's preferences and interests with others.

4.3 Explain how to challenge discrimination and oppressive practice of others when working with an individual with dementia.

? Reflect

How do you involve carers in the care and support of individuals with dementia? Think about your recent contact with carers and the extent to which you have formed positive relationships with them.

- involving them in all aspects of planning support and care
- forming positive relationships with carers
- treating carers respectfully and working in partnership with them to ensure the individual's needs are met appropriately
- using a person-centred approach that acknowledges and respects the individuality and specific needs and preferences of the person with dementia
- encouraging and supporting carers so that they allow the individual to have control and make decisions about care and daily living activities
- modelling good practice in the ways you communicate with and provide care for individuals with dementia
- providing factsheets and other sources of information on issues concerning carers
- helping carers to make links to others in carer support groups
- sharing ideas about care provision and suggestions for activities that would engage the individual who has dementia.

People who care for partners and relatives with dementia tend to be very committed to providing high quality care and support. Most people in this situation will need support and help themselves, at some point. This might include help to provide care so that carers can have some time off, or emotional support to express their feelings and concerns about the situation they are dealing with. Health and social care workers can play an important role in enabling carers to acknowledge, look for and obtain the kinds of support they need.

 Investigate

Ask the manager of your care setting or a senior colleague about the ways in which carers and relatives of individuals with dementia are provided with support by your care organisation. Are there any carers' meetings or a support group for carer's to meet each other and chat to staff members, for example?

Practical Assessment Task

This assessment task covers DEM 313 4.1, 4.2, 4.3.

Health and social care workers need to be able to work with carers and a variety of other colleagues in order to provide effective care for individuals with dementia. These relationships provide an opportunity for health and social care workers to promote diversity and equality and to challenge discrimination and oppressive practice in relation to dementia care. In this activity you are required to show that you can do the following:

1. *work with others to promote diversity and equality for individuals with dementia*

2. *demonstrate how to share the individual's preferences and interests with others*

3. *explain how to challenge discrimination and the oppressive practice of others when working with an individual with dementia.*

Your evidence must be based on your practice in a real work environment and must be witnessed by or be in a format acceptable to your assessor.

Assessment checklist

The knowledge-based assessment criteria for DEM 310, DEM 304 and DEM 313 are listed in the 'What you need to know' table below and on page 124. The practical or competence-based criteria for DEM 304 and DEM 313 are listed in the 'What you need to do' table on pages 124 and 125. Your tutor or assessor will help you to prepare for your assessment, and the tasks suggested in the chapter will help you to create the evidence that you need.

Assessment criteria	What you need to know	Assessment task
DEM 310		
1.1	Explain what is meant by the terms diversity, anti-discriminatory practice and anti-oppressive practice	Page 85
1.2	Explain why it is important to recognise and respect an individual's heritage	Page 85
1.3	Describe why an individual with dementia may be subjected to discrimination and oppression	Page 85
1.4	Describe how discrimination and oppressive practice can be challenged	Page 85
2.1	Explain why it is important to identify an individual's specific and unique needs	Page 96
2.2	Compare the experience of dementia for an individual who has acquired it as an older person with the experience of an individual who has acquired it as a younger person	Page 88
2.3	Describe how the experience of an individual's dementia may impact on carers	Page 88
2.4	Describe how the experience of dementia may be different for individuals who have a learning disability, who are from different ethnic backgrounds, or who are at the end of life	Page 92
3.1	Explain how current legislation and government policy supports person-centred working	Page 104
3.2	Explain how person-centred working can ensure that an individual's specific and unique needs are met	Page 96
3.3	Describe ways of helping an individual's carers or others understand the principles of person-centred care	Page 96
3.4	Identify practical ways of helping the individual with dementia maintain their identity	Page 96

Assessment criteria	What you need to know	Assessment task
DEM 304		
1.1	Explain the impact of key legislation that relates to fulfilment of rights and choices and the minimising of risk of harm for an individual with dementia	Page 104
1.2	Evaluate agreed ways of working that relate to rights and choices of an individual with dementia	Page 106
1.3	Explain how and when personal information may be shared with carers and others taking into account legislative frameworks and agreed ways of working	Page 106
DEM 313		
1.1	Explain why it is important to recognise and respect an individual's heritage	Page 85
1.2	Compare the experience of dementia for an individual who has acquired it as an older person with the experience of an individual who has acquired it as a younger person	Page 88
1.3	Describe how the experience of dementia may be different for individuals who have a learning disability, who are from different ethnic backgrounds or who are at the end of life	Page 92
1.4	Describe how the experience of an individual's dementia may impact on carers	Page 88
2.1	Describe how current legislation, government policy and agreed ways of working support inclusive practice for dementia care and support	Page 104
2.2	Describe the ways in which an individual with dementia may be subjected to discrimination and oppression	Page 85
2.3	Explain the potential impact of discrimination on an individual with dementia	Page 85
2.4	Analyse how diversity, equality and inclusion are addressed in dementia care and support	Page 85
Assessment criteria	**What you need to do**	**Assessment task**
DEM 304		
2.1	Demonstrate that the best interests of an individual with dementia are considered when planning and delivering care and support	Page 112
2.2	Demonstrate how an individual with dementia can be enabled to exercise their rights and choices even when a decision has not been deemed to be in their best interests	Page 112

Assessment criteria	What you need to do	Assessment task
DEM 304		
2.3	Explain why it is important not to assume that an individual with dementia cannot make their own decisions	Page 112
2.4	Describe how the ability of an individual with dementia to make decisions may fluctuate	Page 112
3.1	Demonstrate how carers and others can be involved in planning support that promotes the rights and choices of an individual with dementia and minimises risk of harm	Page 120
3.2	Describe how a conflict of interest can be addressed between the carer and an individual with dementia while balancing rights, choices and risks	Page 120
3.3	Describe how to ensure an individual with dementia, carers and others feel able to complain without fear of retribution	Page 120
4.1	Describe how to maintain privacy and dignity when providing personal support for intimate care to an individual with dementia	Page 116
4.2	Demonstrate that key physical aspects of the environment are enabling care workers to show respect and dignity for an individual with dementia	Page 116
4.3	Demonstrate that key social aspects of the environment are enabling care workers to show respect and dignity for an individual with dementia	Page 116
DEM 313		
3.1	Demonstrate how to identify an individual's uniqueness	Page 98
3.2	Demonstrate how to use life experiences and circumstances of an individual who has dementia to ensure their inclusion	Page 98
3.3	Demonstrate practical ways of helping an individual with dementia to maintain their dignity	Page 98
3.4	Demonstrate how to engage and include an individual with dementia in daily life	Page 98
4.1	Work with others to promote diversity and equality for individuals with dementia	Page 122
4.2	Demonstrate how to share the individual's preferences and interests with others	Page 122
4.3	Explain how to challenge discrimination and oppressive practice of others when working with an individual with dementia	Page 122

4 | The use of medication in dementia care

DEM 305
LO1 Understand the common medications available to, and appropriate for, individuals with dementia

- ▶ Outline the most common medications used to treat symptoms of dementia

- ▶ Describe how commonly-used medications affect individuals with dementia

- ▶ Explain the risks and benefits of anti-psychotic medication for individuals with dementia

- ▶ Explain the importance of recording and reporting side effects/adverse reactions to medication

- ▶ Describe how 'as required' (PRN) medication can be used to support individuals with dementia who may be in pain

DEM 305
LO2 Understand how to provide person-centred care to individuals with dementia through the appropriate and effective use of medication

- ▶ Describe person-centred ways of administering medicines while adhering to administration instructions

- ▶ Explain the importance of advocating for an individual with dementia who may be prescribed medication

HSC 3047
LO1 Understand the legislative framework for the use of medication in social care settings

- ▶ Identify legislation that governs the use of medication in social care settings

- ▶ Outline the legal classification system for medication

- ▶ Explain how and why policies and procedures or agreed ways of working must reflect and incorporate legislative requirements

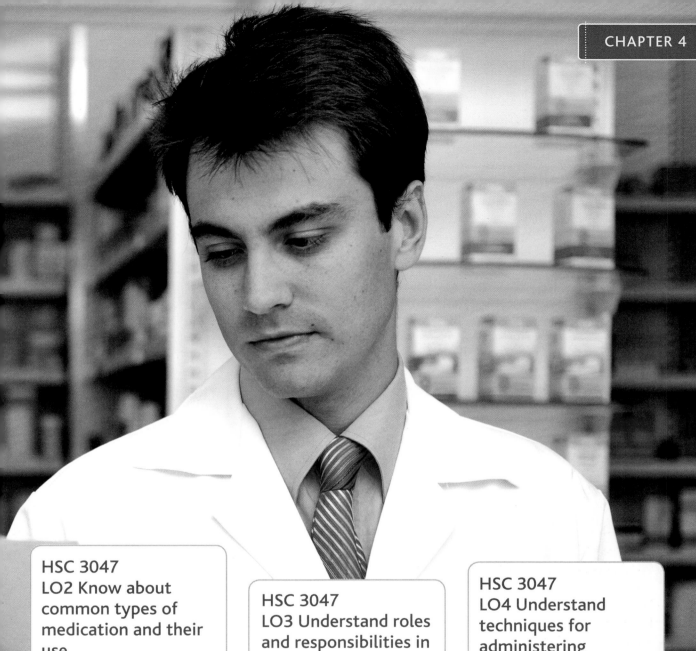

**HSC 3047
LO2 Know about common types of medication and their use**

▶ Identify common types of medication

▶ List conditions for which each type of medication may be prescribed

▶ Describe changes to an individual's physical or mental wellbeing that may indicate an adverse reaction to a medication

**HSC 3047
LO3 Understand roles and responsibilities in the use of medication in social care settings**

▶ Describe the roles and responsibilities of those involved in prescribing, dispensing and supporting use of medication

▶ Explain where responsibilities lie in relation to use of 'over the counter' remedies and supplements

**HSC 3047
LO4 Understand techniques for administering medication**

▶ Describe the routes by which medication can be administered

▶ Describe different forms in which medication may be presented

▶ Describe materials and equipment that can assist in administering medication

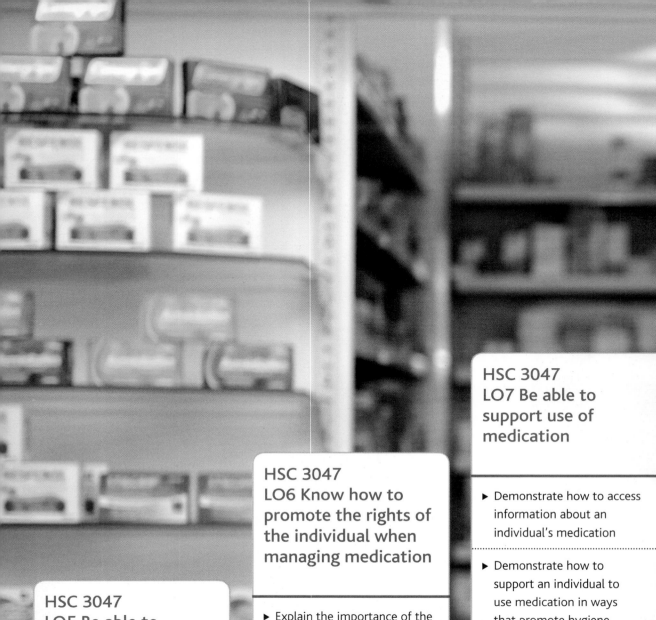

**HSC 3047
LO5 Be able to
receive, store and
dispose of medication
supplies safely**

▶ Demonstrate how to receive
supplies of medication in line
with agreed ways of working

▶ Demonstrate how to store
medication safely

▶ Demonstrate how to dispose
of unused or unwanted
medication safely

**HSC 3047
LO6 Know how to
promote the rights of
the individual when
managing medication**

▶ Explain the importance of the
following principles in the use
of medication:
  • consent
  • self-medication or active
    participation
  • dignity and privacy
  • confidentiality

▶ Explain how risk assessment
can be used to promote an
individual's independence in
managing medication

▶ Describe how ethical issues
that may arise over the use of
medication can be addressed

**HSC 3047
LO7 Be able to
support use of
medication**

▶ Demonstrate how to access
information about an
individual's medication

▶ Demonstrate how to
support an individual to
use medication in ways
that promote hygiene,
safety, dignity and active
participation

▶ Demonstrate strategies to
ensure that medication is used
or administered correctly

▶ Demonstrate how to address
any practical difficulties that
may arise when medication
is used

▶ Demonstrate how and when
to access further information
or support about the use
of medication

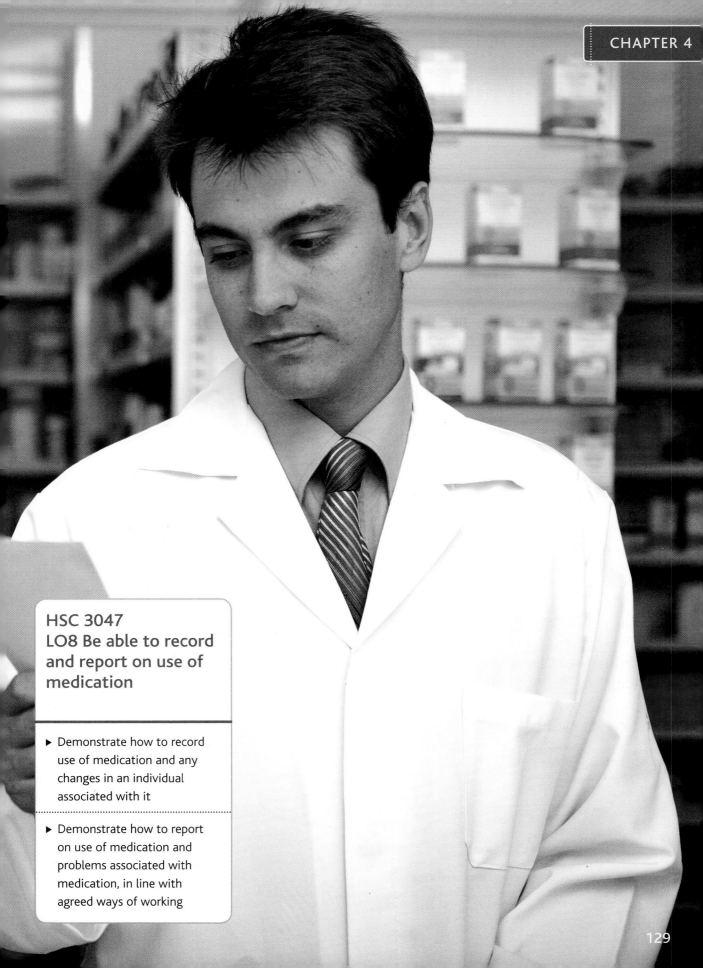

HSC 3047
LO8 Be able to record and report on use of medication

▶ Demonstrate how to record use of medication and any changes in an individual associated with it

▶ Demonstrate how to report on use of medication and problems associated with medication, in line with agreed ways of working

Understand the legislative framework for the use of medication in social care settings

Your assessment criteria:

HSC 3047

1.1 Identify legislation that governs the use of medication in social care settings.

1.2 Outline the legal classification system for medication.

1.3 Explain how and why policies and procedures or agreed ways of working must reflect and incorporate legislative requirements.

The term 'legislative framework' refers to the law that governs different aspects of care. Everyone is subject to the law. In health and social care, the law stipulates what care providers should do and what they cannot do. In social care settings, one of the things that the law or the legislative framework governs is the use of medication. The legislative framework dictates what practitioners should do with respect to the use of medication and what they should not do.

There are a number of laws that are aimed at the use and misuse of drugs and medications. The Misuse of Drugs Act (1971) is intended to prevent the non-medical use of certain drugs. These drugs are known as controlled drugs and some can be found in use in social care settings. These include barbiturates, steroids and some tranquilisers. However, the laws that are most likely to affect the use of medication in social care and other settings where individual are living with dementia are:

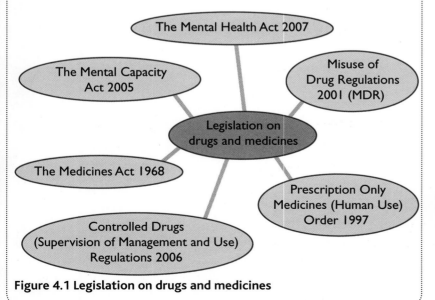

Figure 4.1 Legislation on drugs and medicines

- The Mental Health Act 2007
- The Mental Capacity Act 2005
- Misuse of Drug Regulations 2001 (MDR)
- Legislation on drugs and medicines
- The Medicines Act 1968
- Controlled Drugs (Supervision of Management and Use) Regulations 2006
- Prescription Only Medicines (Human Use) Order 1997

Key terms

Controlled drugs: a prescription medicine containing a drug that is controlled under the Misuse of Drugs legislation to prevent misuse, harm and being obtained illegally

Medication: a chemical substance used as a medicine to cure, treat or prevent disease

Reflect

Reflect on the types of medicines and other remedies and supplements you have used. How did you get them? Were they prescribed or did you buy them 'over the counter'?

The Medicines Act 1968

This law governs the manufacture and supply of medicine, and affects medications bought at the pharmacist, those prescribed by a doctor and any medicine that is commonly available in many shops and online. It divides medicines into three categories.

1. *Prescription only medicines (POMs)*. These are restricted and cannot be bought in pharmacies or other shops. They can only be sold or supplied by a pharmacist if prescribed by a doctor. An example is a course of antibiotics, which must be prescribed by a doctor. They should only be administered to the individual to whom they are prescribed.

2. *Pharmacy medicines*. These can be sold without a prescription, but only by a pharmacist. An example of a medicine that comes into this category is an inhaler used for hay fever.

3. *General Sales List medicines*. General Sales List medicines can be sold by any shop, not just a pharmacy. Examples are common painkillers such as Paracetamol and Nurofen. However, there are restrictions on the advertising, labelling and production of these medicines. Paracetamol, for instance, can only be bought in limited quantities.

In a social care setting, a worker should not buy medication for any individual in their care. You do not know if it might interact with other medicines the person is taking, or if the individual has an adverse reaction to it.

The Prescription Only Medicines (Human Use) Order 1997

This law lists all the prescription-only medicines (POMs) and who can prescribe them. It provides clarity about the category that any medicine falls in. This is important as it is then possible to differentiate between POMs, pharmacy medicines and General Sales List medicines.

The Controlled Drugs (Supervision of Management and Use) Regulations 2006

The management of controlled drugs falls under the Misuse of Drugs Act (1971). The Controlled Drugs (Supervision of Management and Use) Regulations provide the legislative framework for the control and regulation of controlled drugs. Controlled drugs are medicines that can be prescribed under certain conditions, usually for pain relief.

? Reflect

Think about common medicines you are familiar with. What medicine category do they belong in?

Investigate

When you next go shopping, examine the general sales medicines that are for sale in shops. What are the most common and what are they remedies for?

The regulations stipulate how the medicines are to be stored so that they cannot be easily accessed by unauthorised people or confused with other categories of drugs (for instance, by being stored in the same place).

The Misuse of Drugs Regulations 2001

The Misuse of Drugs Regulations (2001) govern the use of dangerous and controlled drugs. They make the storage, use and recording of certain medicines extremely important if workers want to avoid the charge of being a drug dealer!

Reflect

Why do you think controlled drugs are governed by additional legislation? To what extent should they be subject to special measures to control their availability?

Investigate

Investigate policies, procedures and agreed ways of working with respect to medication management where you work.

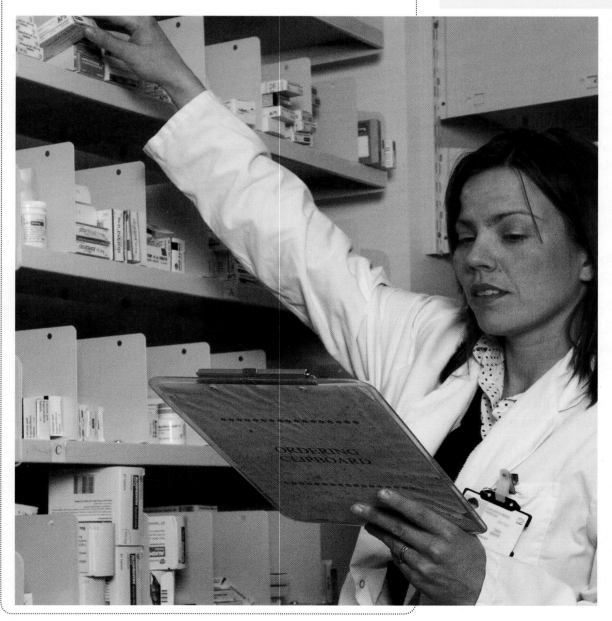

The Mental Health Act 2007

The Mental Health Act (2007) provides for the care and treatment of individuals with mental health problems. Individuals might live in the community or reside in social care settings. In certain circumstances the Act allows doctors to treat individuals for a mental health problem even if the individual does not want to be treated. The treatment is often in the form of medication taken as tablets or as an injection. You should be aware if the individual in your care is subject to a section of the Mental Health Act.

The Mental Capacity Act 2005

This Act aims to protect the interests of individuals who are deemed not to have mental capacity – that is, they are not able to make informed decisions about how they should be cared for. It usually applies to older people with dementia, but other individuals might be subject to the Act. It must be assumed that any individual has the capacity to make their own decisions, unless it is established that the individual lacks capacity. This means the individual should be allowed to decide if they want to take medication, based on sufficient information that allows them to make an informed choice. In a social care setting the individual cannot be compelled to take medication even if the prescriber thinks it is in their best interest to do so, if that individual does not wish to take the medicine.

How and why must practices reflect the legislative requirements?

Policies and procedures and other agreed ways of working must reflect and incorporate the legislative framework because:

- it contributes to the safety of individuals who take medicines as well as other people

- it ensures that the individual has access to the appropriate treatment

- it enables differentiation between different categories of medicines and their use

- it is against the law not to comply with the legislative framework that governs the provision of medicines in social care settings.

Policies and procedures and other agreed ways of working must reflect and incorporate the legislative framework by:

- ensuring the safe and appropriate storage of each category of medicine in line with the legislative framework and regulations

Key term

Mental capacity: the ability to make decisions for yourself

- having suitably trained members of staff to prescribe and administer medicines in the required way

- having measures in place to supervise and check the safe ordering, storage and recording of all prescription-only and other medicines.

Case study – legislation and policies

Amanda, who was completing a placement at a residential home for people with dementia, was asked by a resident's close relative for information about how she could acquire the medicines her mother was given. The relative wanted to take her mother, Mary, who had been in the home for a month, to another home closer to her family.

At first Amanda did not understand what the relative was asking for. The relative did not seem to realise that the medication was prescribed by doctors. The relative said she assumed that the care workers at the home went to the pharmacist in town to buy drugs for the residents. Amanda explained that it was not possible to buy all the medication used and that the use of medication is governed by legislation.

1. Name three pieces of legislation that control the use of medicines.

2. How are medicines classified under the Medicines Act 1968?

3. What could Amanda tell the relative about medicines that are available to buy at the pharmacist?

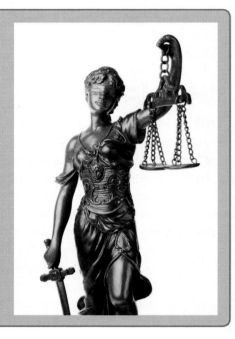

Knowledge Assessment Task

This assessment task covers HSC 3047 1.1, 1.2, 1.3.

It is important that care workers understand the legislative framework that governs what they do, and this includes laws about the use of medication. In this knowledge assessment task you are required to show that you understand the legislative framework for the use of medication in social care settings.

Imagine you are responsible for training where you work. You are asked to design a training booklet about medication use. The booklet should contain information that:

1. *identifies legislation that governs the use of medication in social care settings*

2. *identifies the legal classification systems for medication*

3. *explains policies and procedures in place in your work area that reflect and incorporate legislative requirements.*

Design the booklet.

 Discuss

Discuss with your line manager how local policies and legislative requirements are complied with in your work setting.

Understand the common medications available to, and appropriate for, individuals with dementia, and their use

To work safely with people living with dementia, practitioners must understand the medications that individuals receive. Workers' awareness should include knowledge about the common types of medications used and why they are prescribed to individuals with dementia. They should be especially aware of the risks and benefits to individuals with dementia who use anti-psychotic medicines. Risks might include adverse changes to a person's mental or physical wellbeing, necessitating accurate recording and reporting of side-effects. As required (PRN) medication is also sometimes necessary, for instance if an individual is in pain.

Common types of medication used to treat individuals with dementia

The most commonly used medications affecting individuals with dementia are:

- medications that manage multi-infarct dementia – dementia resulting from repeated small strokes that lead to damage to the surrounding brain tissue

- medications that help manage subcortical dementias – benign or harmless tumours and hydrocephalus

- medications that offer neuroprotection – that is, protection against further damage – and enhance cognitive ability.

Many older people in health and social care have a cognitive impairment with a type of dementia. While they may have memory problems, they can also experience other symptoms associated with mental health problems such as feeling depressed or having strange and disturbing psychotic experiences. In fact, more people have depression than dementia, and having dementia does not exclude an individual from being depressed as well.

The table on the next page (figure 4.2) outlines a sample of the main types of medicine, names of specific drugs and their use in treating the symptoms of dementia. The generic drug name is given with the UK trade name in brackets.

Your assessment criteria:

DEM 305

1.1 Outline the most common medications used to treat symptoms of dementia.

1.2 Describe how commonly-used medications affect individuals with dementia.

1.3 Explain the risks and benefits of anti-psychotic medication for individuals with dementia.

HSC 3047

2.1 Identify common types of medication.

2.2 List conditions for which each type of medication may be prescribed.

2.3 Describe changes to an individual's physical or mental wellbeing that may indicate an adverse reaction to a medication.

Investigate

Which colleagues in your work setting are able to administer medication? What qualifications do they have?

Key terms

Hydrocephalus: a build-up of fluids in the skull that leads to brain swelling

PRN: an abbreviation of the Latin phrase pro re nata, *meaning in the circumstances or as circumstances arise, used for medicine given as required - instead of on a regular basis*

Figure 4.2 Medication to treat dementia

Type of medicine	Examples of specific drugs	Symptom it is used to treat
Cognitive enhancement and neuroprotection	Donepezil Hydrochloride (Aricept) Galantamine (Reminyl) Rivastigmine (Exelon) Memantine (EBIXA)	Mild to moderate Alzheimer dementia including: short-term memory loss, apathy and lack of motivation Moderate to severe dementia including: loss of memory, poor motivation, confusion and disorientation
Anti-psychotic medication/ neuroleptics	Olanzapine (Zyprexa) Amisulpiride (Solian) Risperidone (Risperdal) Haloperidol (Haldol) Zuclopenthixol (Clopixol) Chlorpromazine (Largactil)	Hearing voices, paranoid ideas delusional and strange beliefs, disrupted thinking
Anti-depressant medication	Doxepine (Sinequan) Citalopram (Cipramil) Fluoxetine (Prozac) Paroxetine (Seroxat) Venlafaxine (Efexor) Mirtazapine (Zispin) Trazodone (Molipaxin) Lofepramine (Gamanil) Amitriptyline (Tryptizol)	Loss of energy and interest, sadness, poor concentration and altered appetite and sleep patterns

What changes to an individual's wellbeing may indicate an adverse reaction to medication?

Individuals can have adverse reactions to any medication, not only those that are used in health and social care settings. The type and severity of effect depends on the medication that is used and the tolerance of the individual to that medicine.

The table opposite illustrates common adverse effects to named medications. While this is not an exhaustive list of medications in each group, they do indicate typical adverse reactions that each category of medicine might cause. It is important that you find out what medication each individual you are looking after is prescribed, and familiarise yourself with the type of adverse effects they may experience.

 Discuss

What adverse reactions to medication have occurred in your care setting? How are they identified through signs and symptoms, and what special actions should be taken in response to them, if any?

Figure 4.3 Common adverse reactions to medications

Type of medicine	Common adverse reactions
Cognitive enhancers including: Donepezil (Aricept), Galantamine (Reminyl) and Rivastigmine (Exelon)	Nausea, vomiting, diarrhoea, insomnia and headache
Anti-psychotics including: Olanzapine (Zyprexa), Amisulpiride (Solian) and Risperidone (Risperdal)	Stiffness, abnormal movements, restlessness, weight gain, apathy and sedation
Anti-depressants including: Doxepine (Sinequan), Citalopram (Cipramil) and Fluoxetine (Prozac)	Sedation, sweating, urinary difficulties, blurred vision, rashes and nausea

Risks and benefits of anti-psychotic medication

Anti-psychotic medication is prescribed for some people with dementia because they experience feelings and thoughts similar to the experiences of people with severe mental health issues. These experiences include thinking that their treasured possessions have been stolen when in reality they have been mislaid or hidden by the individual during a period of confusion. The individual might hear voices, for example believing someone is speaking to them when there is nobody there. Other common symptoms include: strange beliefs, such as that they are being poisoned or thinking the TV or radio is speaking to them personally. These strange ideas can cause distress to the individual and may lead them to behave oddly or out of character. Anti-psychotic medication can reduce or eliminate these distressing symptoms.

However, there are risks to taking anti-psychotic medication. These medications, like all other types of medicine, have side effects. These side effects can raise the risk of misuse of medication – as the side effects include sedation, there is a risk that this kind of medication can be used to quieten down individuals if, for instance, they wander or are noisy or disruptive. The result is over-sedation, a reduction in the quality of life of the individual, which in turn can lead to other physical and psychological problems. Not least among these is similarity between the effects of the misuse of anti-psychotic medication and the symptoms of dementia, in particular apathy and memory problems.

Another side effect to the use of anti-psychotics that puts older people at particular risk is hypotension – a lowering of blood pressure. **Postural hypotension** is a fall in blood pressure when a person stands after lying down or sitting for a long time. This can lead to falls and the older person damaging weakened bone or tissue.

Key term

Postural hypotension: a drop in blood pressure due to a change in body position when a person moves to a more vertical position – from sitting to standing or from lying down to sitting or standing

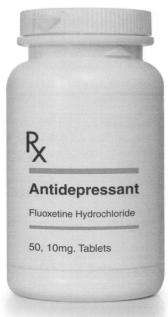

Understand common medications

Case study – common types of medication

Parker has Alzheimer's disease, a type of dementia that has affected his memory, leaving him confused about where he is and who other people are. Lately his wife, Angela, rang their doctor and asked him to visit them. She said that Parker had recently hidden the car keys under the mattress and then accused her of taking them so she could give the car to a young man she knew. In fact, the car had been sold months before when Parker was first told he should not drive any more. The keys were spare from another car they had kept from years before and Angela only gave them to Parker because he kept looking for keys.

While Angela was used to Parker's poor memory and confusion, she found it most difficult when he complained about the young people in the next room talking about him. At times he would shout and say he knew that she planned to leave him for the young man she kept inviting into the house.

1. Name two types of medication the doctor might want to prescribe for Parker.

2. What adverse side effects to the medication would you inform Angela and Parker about?

3. How could anti-psychotic medication help Parker?

4. What risks might there be associated with anti-psychotic medication?

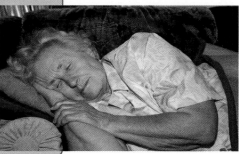

 Reflect

Individuals with dementia often demonstrate signs of other conditions such as depression or psychosis. Reflect on ways you might identify if an individual is depressed or psychotic in addition to having dementia.

Knowledge Assessment Task

This assessment task covers DEM 305 1.1, 1.2, 1.3 and HSC 3047 2.1, 2.2, 2.3.

An understanding of the use and effects of common types of medication will help you support individuals with dementia and contribute to safe and effective practice. In this knowledge assessment task you are required to show that you know about common types of medication and their use with individuals with dementia.

While working in a social care setting with individuals with dementia you are asked by three families, each of which has a relative you are supporting, to give them information about the medication their relative is using.

What would you tell each family about a common type of medication, the conditions it is prescribed for, and any potential adverse reactions?

Family 1 – the relative has dementia and has psychotic experiences

Family 2 – the relative has dementia and is being treated for depression

Family 3 – the relative has dementia

Record your answers in a way acceptable to your assessor.

 Discuss

Discuss with colleagues where you work the risks and benefits of medication. Do colleagues think that it is always better to take medication, or do the risks outweigh any benefit to the individual?

 Investigate

All medications have adverse reactions or side effects. Using the BNF (British National Formulary) or BNF online, investigate the side effects to cognitive enhancers such as Aricept, Reminyl and Exelon.

Roles and responsibilities involved in use of medication

While each professional and care worker in social care settings has a duty of care towards individuals they look after, they also have specific roles and responsibilities. These specific roles and responsibilities extend to prescribing, dispensing and supporting the use of medication. Note how care support workers have duties with respect to medication, reflecting their role as working more closely with the individual.

The table below illustrates the key roles and responsibilities of professionals and workers in social care with respect to medication.

Your assessment checklist:

HSC 3047

3.1 Describe the roles and responsibilities of those involved in prescribing, dispensing and supporting use of medication.

3.2 Explain where responsibilities lie in relation to use of 'over the counter' remedies and supplements.

Figure 4.4 Roles and responsibilities regarding medication

Title	Role	Key responsibilities
Doctor	To examine the individual and diagnose their health condition or illness To prescribe treatment that might include medication to treat the condition or illness To reassess if the treatment for the condition or illness has been effective To liaise closely with the individual or persons caring for the individual	To ensure that the individual's health status is determined and interventions instigated and monitored
Pharmacist	To confirm that any medication treatment is not going to harm the individual, including the correct dose and means of administration To make the medication available in the correct quantity with instructions for the safe use of the medication To pack the medication in a suitable format, for instance in a dosette box (see overleaf), easy-peel wrapping or other container	To ensure the safe dispensing of medication to the individual or those caring for the individual
Care worker	To communicate with the doctor and pharmacist regarding the medication To ensure the medication is available for the individual as prescribed by the doctor To store the medication safely, complying with local and national guidelines To administer the medication to the individual in the correct dose and by the correct method of administration, or ensure that the individual takes the medication safely as prescribed To observe for adverse reactions and side effects to the medication To dispose of any residual materials safely To record the administration of the medication To monitor the individual's condition or health status	To ensure the safe storage, administration, recording and disposal of medication

While the care worker has specific roles and responsibilities in the administration of medication, as listed on the previous page they also have responsibilities to ensure the individual gives consent to receive medication.

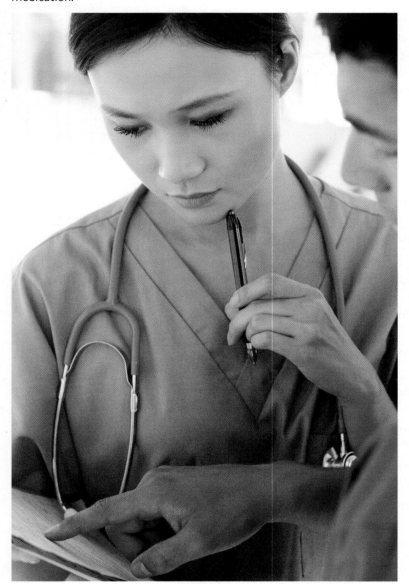

'Over the counter' remedies and supplements

'Over the counter' remedies and supplements are widely available in shops and supermarkets. They can be bought by adults over the age of 18 as remedies for the symptoms of colds or other common ailments, and analgesia for headaches and pains.

Read the case study on the next page, and then answer the questions that follow.

Case study

Annie likes to help people. This was one of the reasons she chose a career in social care; there are plenty of opportunities to help and support people in lots of different ways. Mrs Abel (79), whom Annie has got to know quite well from her care work in Meadowside Residential Home, often talks to Annie about what she does when she is not on duty. One day Mrs Abel asks Annie, saying it is because she is so helpful and kind, to get her some vitamin and mineral supplements from a well-known chemist store on the way home. She then offers Annie a £10 note to buy them. Annie feels flattered that Mrs Abel thinks she is helpful and kind; it makes Annie feel good to hear it. She does not like saying 'no' to anyone.

1. What should Annie do?

2. Why should she do this?

Investigate

What policies are in place in your work setting (if any) that concern the relationships between the cared for and the caregivers? Why is it important that people with dementia should be protected from some relationships?

In this case study Annie is put in an awkward position by Mrs Abel. She wants to help her. She should, though, bear in mind the following:

1. Annie does not know what other medication Mrs Abel takes or how the vitamin and mineral supplements would interact with other medication.

2. Has Mrs Abel asked anyone else to do the same errand?

3. What is the policy of Meadowside for residents keeping their own source of medication or other remedies?

4. What is the policy of Meadowside for boundaries of relationships between members of staff and residents?

5. Is it a breach of the guidelines on the administration of medication?

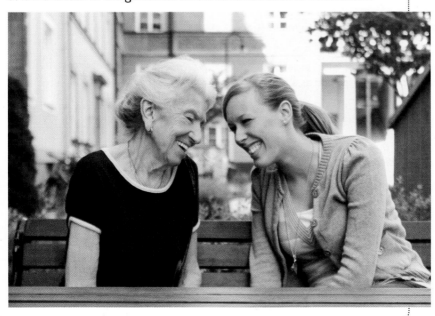

Fortunately Annie realises that she should not buy 'over the counter' remedies or supplements for Mrs Abel – or any other resident. She knows that she would be held responsible should there be any adverse reaction with this older person.

Having reflected on the situation later with her line manager, Annie realises that responsibilities do not just lie with her.

- Meadowside has a responsibility to maintain the safety of all their residents and staff. What would happen if another resident got hold of the supplements and consumed them?

- Meadowside has a responsibility to comply with national and local standards for the safe storage of all medicines including remedies and supplements.

- Meadowside has a responsibility to ensure that care workers are familiar with the policies on medication and its management.

- Annie has a responsibility to maintain the safety of all residents within her capabilities.

- Annie has a responsibility to comply with known national and local policies.

Reflect

Usually there are many professionals and workers who are involved in the care of an individual with dementia. Of all these people, who has the role and responsibility to ensure that day-to-day medication management is person-centred?

Investigate

Investigate the policy for medication management where you work. What does it say about using a person-centred approach to medication management?

Discuss

Discuss with your line manager about how the care setting where you work communicates with outside practitioners involved in medication management.

Knowledge Assessment Task

This assessment task covers HSC 3047 3.1, 3.2.

There are many roles carried out by a range of professionals and workers in social care, and care workers should be aware of the responsibilities other practitioners carry. In this knowledge assessment task you are required to show that you understand the roles of others with respect to medication management.

You are asked to depict key roles and responsibilities with respect to medication management as a poster that can be displayed as a reminder for members of staff.

Design a poster that:

1. *describes the roles and responsibilities of those involved in prescribing, dispensing and supporting the use of medication*

2. *explains where responsibilities lie with respect to 'over the counter' remedies and supplements.*

Discuss your ideas for the poster with your assessor before you begin to design it.

Techniques for the administration of medication

Medication comes in different forms and can be administered by a range of means and routes. Special materials and equipment might also be required. As a care worker it is necessary to know about the different routes through which medication can be given, the different forms it may be presented in, and the materials and equipment that might be needed to assist when administering medication.

The routes by which medication can be administered are shown in the table below.

Figure 4.5 Routes to administer medication

Route	Description
Oral or by mouth	This is the most common route for the administration of medication. Tablets, capsules, lozenges and other pills are taken orally, as well as syrups and other medicinal fluids
	Some inhalers are taken orally, such as with asthma
Gastrostomy tube	A gastrostomy tube may be used if it is already in place and the person cannot take anything by mouth
Sublingual or under the tongue	A lozenge is placed under the tongue for quick absorption
Subcutaneous or under the skin	This is by the means of a needle, which is placed under the skin to administer medication in fluid form
Intramuscular or in the muscle	This route involves a needle piercing the skin to administer medication deep into the muscle. This is often given in the gluteus maximus or buttock, or in the upper arm
Anal or rectal	A medication in the form of a suppository is inserted into the rectum
Optical or in the eye	Drops are placed in the eye(s)
Aural or in the ear	Drops are placed in the ear(s)
Topical or on the surface	Creams or lotions are applied to the skin
Nasal or via the nose	Hay fever sprays are an example
Nasogastric tube	A nasogastric tube may be used for some medication if it is in place and the person cannot take anything by mouth

As well as being administered via a range of routes, medication can be presented in different forms:

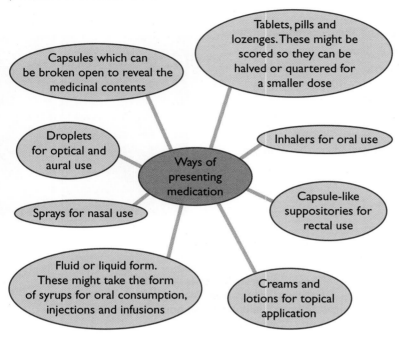

Figure 4.6 Ways of presenting medication

Diagram nodes:
- Capsules which can be broken open to reveal the medicinal contents
- Tablets, pills and lozenges. These might be scored so they can be halved or quartered for a smaller dose
- Droplets for optical and aural use
- Ways of presenting medication
- Inhalers for oral use
- Sprays for nasal use
- Capsule-like suppositories for rectal use
- Fluid or liquid form. These might take the form of syrups for oral consumption, injections and infusions
- Creams and lotions for topical application

Some medication can be administered comparatively simply, for instance as a tablet taken from a plastic bottle. However, some medications require special equipment if they are to be administered properly and safely.

Material and equipment to assist in administering medication

The material and equipment used when administering medication depends on the technique and route of administration. A single tablet administered in a health or social care setting requires a small medicine cup to transfer the tablet between the person giving the medicine and the person receiving the medicine. This is to ensure the tablet remains safe and clean. Medication administered by injection, on the other hand, requires specialist equipment to make sure it is administered in an appropriate and safe way.

Materials can refer to an assemblage of items such as antiseptic swabs, gauze and plasters, trays and medicine pots, and dosette boxes that aid the administration of medication, whereas equipment might refer to the tools that are used, such as syringes, needles and ampoules.

Investigate

With the permission of your line manager/supervisor, find out all the ways of presenting medicines in your work setting. Which are the most frequently used ways to give medicines?

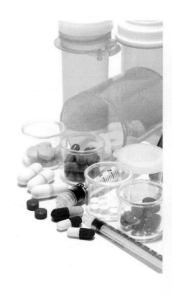

Syringes

A **syringe** is a piece of equipment used with a needle to administer parenteral medication by injection. Parenteral means that it does not make use of the digestive or respiratory system as a tablet would. Injections can be given intramuscularly (into the muscle), subcutaneously (below the skin), intravenously (into a vein) and intradermally (into the skin). Of these, the first two are the most likely to be encountered in a social care setting; intramuscular injections are given as inoculations and to relieve psychotic symptoms, for example, and insulin is injected where the individual has diabetes using a subcutaneous injection.

There are several types of syringe, differing in shape and size and made from different materials. Each syringe has three parts: the barrel or outside part, the plunger which fits inside the barrel and the tip where the needle is connected. The types of syringe include:

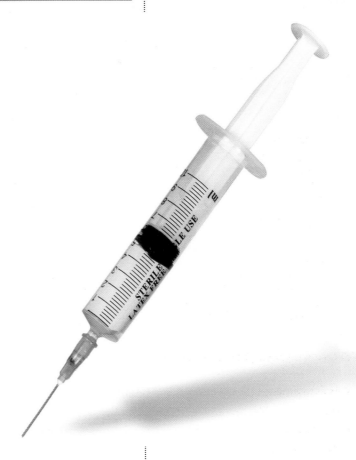

- hypodermic syringe with a millilitre scale marked on the barrel

- insulin syringe that has a scale specially designed for insulin

- prefilled unit-dose systems that are ready for use or a prefilled cartridge and needles that needs a reusable holder (injection system) to be attached before use.

Needles and ampoules

Needles are made of stainless steel and are usually disposable due to the risk of cross infection if they are shared or used more than once. They are available in different sizes, usually between 1 and 5 centimetres long and #18–#28 in diameter or **gauge**.

Ampoules and vials are used to carry medication that is to be given by injection. An ampoule is a glass container, with a constricted neck varying in size from 1–20 millilitres or more.

Key terms

Gauge: needles come in different diameters; a needle gauge is derived from the Birmingham Wire Gauge where the smaller gauge numbers refer to larger needle outer diameters

Syringe: a piece of equipment used with a needle to administer an injection

A vial is a small glass bottle with a sealed rubber cap. A needle is used to pierce the vial through the rubber and then changed for a clean needle to inject the individual.

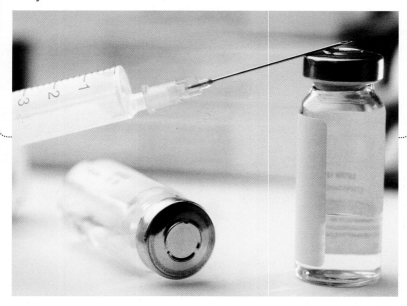

This assessment task covers HSC 3047 4.1, 4.2, 4.3.

Care workers need to understand the techniques used when administering medication as they may be required to assist in medication management. Therefore, it is necessary to know about the different routes through which medication can be given, the different forms it may be presented in, and the materials and equipment that might be needed to assist when administering medication.

In this knowledge assessment task you are required to show that you understand techniques for administering medication.

With the support and permission of your line manager, investigate all the different medications used by individuals in the care setting where you work. For each medication:

1. *identify the route by which it is administered*

2. *identify different forms it can be presented in*

3. *describe materials and equipment that can assist on administering medication*

4. *identify any other forms of medication, routes of administering, materials and equipment that are not used where you work.*

Present your findings in a format acceptable to your assessor.

 Reflect

There are many different ways that medication can be used. Reflect on which techniques you would be most comfortable with if you were prescribed different medications that required different routes to be administered. Why is this?

 Discuss

Discuss with your line manager and colleagues the different techniques and routes of medication management used commonly in your care setting.

Investigate

With the permission of your line manager and the consent of individuals in your care, access prescription administration charts and identify how different medications are administered.

 Key term

Prescription administration chart: *a record of the medicines given to an individual in a care setting*

How to receive, store and dispose of medication supplies safely

When receiving supplies of medication you must always work within policies and ways of working. This is to ensure the security of the medication and everyone's safety.

Read the following case study and then answer the questions that follow.

Case study

Caroline works at Longside Residential Home for older people with dementia and other long-term conditions, for which they need considerable support in activities of everyday living.

One morning she notices the car from the local pharmacy pull up in the grounds of the home and goes to welcome the driver. About this time every week they receive a supply of the medication required by the residents for the coming week. Caroline is pleased to see that it is Davy Jones delivering the medicines. She likes him and the stories he tells about life on the road as he does his delivery round.

Davy enters carrying a locked container with the medication. Caroline greets him and takes him to the back office – the locked room where medicines, syringes and other medical equipment is stored. On the way she shows a confused resident where the day room is. She asks Davy to put the locked medicines transportation container down on the table and then opens it in front of him, looks briefly inside and offers him a coffee. He accepts so they go to the kitchen.

1. In what ways did Caroline neglect to ensure the security of the medication?

2. In what ways did Caroline put others at risk?

It is vital that care workers are aware of local policies and comply with agreed ways of working. In what ways might Caroline not have complied with agreed ways of working?

- She has not shared the information with the Home's manager that the medication has arrived.

- There is no indication that she or anyone else signed to formally receive the medicines.

- The medicines have not been checked or stored correctly.

- She left the medicine box open and unattended.

- She did not lock the door to the back office.

? Reflect

There will be arrangements for medication to be delivered to your work setting. Reflect on how confidentiality and safety can be compromised if proper procedures are not followed.

Investigate

How are medicines ordered and delivered where you work? Who orders them and when? What documentation is used?

How to store medicines safely

All medicines must be stored in a way that complies with local policies. These policies will include:

Medication that is to be taken orally (by mouth) should not be stored with medication that is to be taken by other routes

Storing the medicine in accordance with the **patient information leaflet** and instructions on the label

Policies for medicine storage

Storing the medicine within a locked cupboard inside a locked room

Keys to the room and medicine cupboard should be kept secure

Access to the medication should be limited to people who need access to it for the purpose of their employment

Figure 4.7 Policies for medicine storage

Unused or unwanted medication

Sometimes medicines are unused, for instance when the individual has a change of prescription. Medicines might also be unwanted for other reasons, such as that they are out of date or the individual for whom they were supplied has moved on elsewhere. An individual may also remove consent to receive treatment after, for instance, an injection is drawn up ready for administration, but the individual then refuses to accept it.

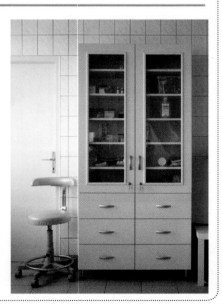

Key term

Patient information leaflet: a small leaflet supplied with medicines that gives details of the medicine, including its use with specific medical conditions, side effects and dosages

Reflect

Why might an individual with dementia refuse their medication?

Whatever the reason the medicines are unused or unwanted, they must be disposed of carefully and with regard to the law.

Unwanted medicines should be returned to a community pharmacy where they can be consigned as medicinal waste, classified as 'household waste' in line with the Controlled Waste Regulations 1992. This includes waste medicines from a person's home and from a residential home.

If a care home also provides nursing care then the community pharmacy cannot accept unwanted medicines as waste. Instead the home must use a licensed waste management company to dispose of the medicine.

- Unwanted or unused medicines should *never* be given to an individual for whom they were not supplied.

- Unwanted or unused medicines should *never* be removed by staff and used for their own purposes.

- Medicine should never be flushed down a toilet.

- Medicines should never be placed in household refuse bins.

In accordance with agreed ways of working, unwanted or unused medicines should be separated from current medicines at the earliest practical opportunity and transported to the community pharmacy or given to the licensed waste management company for disposal.

Reflect

Are there any particular risks with older people with dementia storing their medication at home? How can any risks be minimised?

Discuss

Discuss with your line manager how medications are stored in your work setting. Which medications can be stored together and which should be stored separately? Do any specific medications require refrigeration or room temperature storage? Why is this?

Investigate

Investigate how medications where you work are disposed of. Is a licenced waste company used or are they sent to the community pharmacist? What procedures are followed?

Practical Assessment Task

This assessment task covers HSC 3047 5.1, 5.2, 5.3.

Care workers need to be able to practise safely with respect to medication. This is particularly necessary where individuals have dementia because there are risks present that are different from risks in other client groups. Safe medication management begins with workers being able to receive, store and dispose of medication supplies safely.

For this practical assessment task you are required to demonstrate that you are able to receive, store and dispose of medication supplies safely.

1. *Discuss agreed ways of working on receiving, storing and disposing of medication with your line manager.*

2. *Investigate policies and procedures in your work setting about medication management.*

3. *Demonstrate to your assessor's satisfaction that you can receive, store and dispose of medication safely.*

4. *Provide evidence that you can receive, store and dispose of medication safely as a 300 word written account that includes specific governing legislation.*

Promoting individuals' rights when managing medication

As in other areas of life, individuals have rights in relation to taking medication, and care workers have a duty in upholding these rights. This is particularly so when individuals are vulnerable – for example, when they have dementia. There are actions care workers can carry out that support and promote the rights of individuals while managing medication, and they are important for the reasons explained in the table below.

Your assessment checklist:

HSC 3047

6.1 Explain the importance of the following principles in the use of medication:
  - consent
  - self-medication or active participation
  - dignity and privacy
  - confidentiality.

6.2 Explain how risk assessment can be used to promote an individual's independence in managing medication.

6.3 Describe how ethical issues that may arise over the use of medication can be addressed.

Using risk assessments to promote independence during medication management

Risk assessments on the use of medication are carried out to assess potential and actual risks to individuals concerning medication. The suitability of the medicine is assessed, but so are the means and circumstances in which the medicine is taken. The risk assessment plays an important role in promoting the individual's independence in managing medication.

Read the four vignettes on pages 151–2. They demonstrate different ways that risk assessment promotes the individual's independence in managing medication.

Figure 4.8 Supporting rights when managing medication

Right	Explanation
The right to consent to treatment	That the individual gives permission to be treated is a legal requirement. The process of establishing consent is also one way that care workers can demonstrate that they respect the individual, and is instrumental in developing trust between the care worker and the person being cared for.
The right to actively participate in treatment	Enabling the individual, when it is possible, to actively participate in their treatment through self-medication is important because it helps promote the individual's autonomy and control over their care and treatment.
The right to dignity, privacy and respect	The individual retains their dignity and privacy. This is particularly important when receiving medication that involves a procedure, such as an injection, where clothing is arranged. Privacy is not only one way that care workers can show that they respect the individual, but is also a fundamental human right. The right to privacy is encoded by the articles of the Human Rights Act (1998).
The right to confidentiality	Maintaining confidentiality ensures that the individual's privacy and dignity are not undermined by information about them being shared and discussed by others who have no need to know what medication an individual receives.

Vignette 1

Clarice is 93 years old. She has vascular dementia, but still lives alone in a warden-controlled flat. Twice a day she is supported with taking her medicine. Although she is quite frail, and has rheumatism, the care worker only has to take Clarice's tablets from the packet. Clarice likes a glass of water to help the tablets go down, which she insists on getting herself. However, there are risks involved.

The risk assessment identified walking with a glass of water from the kitchen as a risk, but it is positive risk-taking. It respected Clarice's preferences and promoted her independence with her medication management.

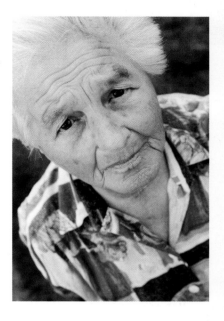

Vignette 2

Sandar is 63 and has an early-onset type of dementia. She does not think there is anything wrong with her, even though she has been behaving oddly – putting the kettle in the oven to boil water and trying to light the electric radiators with a match. She is being assessed for residential care by her social worker. Her husband explains that when it is time for her to have her medicine, a cognitive enhancer called Reminyl, she often refuses. He spends a great deal of time explaining to Sandar what the medicine is for, and why she should take it, before she consents to taking the Reminyl. The social worker notes that there are actual risks to Sandar from her behaviour, and potential risks to her. The risk assessment questions if she being coerced into taking her medication, or whether she needs it for her own good.

Investigate

In what ways does risk assessment where you work contribute to an individual's independence, and how might risk assessment be a barrier to independence?

Because Sandar had presented risks with her behaviour, the risk assessment elements that focused on her medicine management advocated that she should be persuaded to take medicine even if at first she refused. Ultimately this would maintain her level of independence, as otherwise she may have had to be taken into residential care for her own safety.

Vignette 3

Morgan lives in Milkwood, a specialist residential home for older people with dementia. The staff take care of all his everyday needs. His independence in medicine management is promoted after each meal. He likes to help the care staff by clearing some of the tables away before accepting his tablets, but is then reminded and encouraged to collect his medicine from the trolley instead of it being brought to him. In view, though, of his contentment with this arrangement, and his other 'jobs' at the facility, it was decided in consultation with Morgan, and his son, that he should continue clearing the tables away before accepting his tablets.

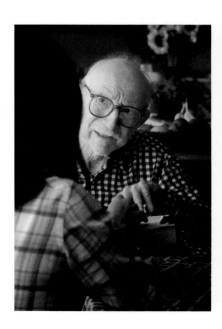

His independence is promoted as he chooses to take the medication when he is ready.

Vignette 4

Rodney has recently been diagnosed with Alzheimer's disease. It is in the early stages and he can continue to live much as he did before his memory started to deteriorate. As a single man, he thought he might have to rely on friends and neighbours for support with his medication. However, it was decided after a risk assessment was carried out that his independence could be promoted and supported if he did as much of the medication management himself for as long as he is able. He collects his prescription from the local chemist who conveniently supplies his cognitive enhancer in weekly packs. This arrangement works well. He is able to self-medicate, checked weekly by the pharmacist.

Each of these vignettes illustrates a way that risk assessments can promote the individual's independence. They should, however, be carried out by a trained worker and in consultation as far as possible with the individual and those who know him or her well.

Ethical issues

Ethics concerns what people do and why they take certain actions. It is a code for behaviour and a branch of moral philosophy that tries to differentiate between what is right and what is wrong.

In social care, and particularly with individuals with dementia, there are a number of ethical issues that affect medication management. Individuals with dementia are vulnerable and often their family carers are vulnerable as well. Therefore great care should be taken to think about the ethics, or what is right and what is wrong, regarding each situation. For instance, dementia can bring with it ethical dilemmas concerning what is the right course of action. Sometimes, what seems the right thing to do in a certain situation may also have harmful effects, and so might be the wrong action.

Typical ethical dilemmas encountered with people with dementia include issues around consent, individual autonomy, confidentiality, iatrogenic adverse effects, beneficence and maleficence and the duty to avoid harm to people you care for.

The table opposite explains some of the ethical issues, and how they might be addressed.

Key terms

Beneficence: *an ethical term meaning that action is taken for the good of others*

Iatrogenesis: *an inadvertent ill effect or adverse reaction to medical treatment*

Maleficence: *the intention to harm others. Non-maleficence is an ethical term that means the intention to avoid doing harm*

Discuss

Ask a colleague to discuss ethical issues they have experienced with individuals with dementia. What was the issue and who was involved? Was there a resolution to the issue and, if so, how was it resolved?

Discuss

Talk with your line manager about the ethical dilemmas they have encountered in the care setting. How were they addressed?

Figure 4.9 Ethical issues surrounding medication of individuals with dementia

Ethical issue	Explanation	Ways it can be addressed
Informed consent	The individual with dementia may not understand why they are offered medicine and as such do not give informed consent for treatment	Frequent explanations of why the medication is prescribed Discussion with family, and other carers, about the individual's preferences with respect to taking medication
Confidentiality	Confidentiality can be breached as others, not just the individual older person, may need to be involved in decisions about medication management	To seek the individual's permission to discuss issues with family and others who know them well
Autonomy	The autonomy or independence of the individual is affected, perhaps by a new reliance on medication	The individual should be encouraged and enabled to participate actively in their own medication management as far as they are able. This includes, if possible, where to have medication, when and in what form
Iatrogenesis	Iatrogenic effects – unintended adverse reactions to medication – can include complex drug reactions as older people are often prescribed more than one medication for a number of health conditions	Medication should be monitored closely and reviewed on a regular basis
Beneficence and maleficence	Care workers have a duty to do good (beneficence) and avoid harming (maleficence) the people they care for. Physiological changes during older age can lead to specific problems including cumulative effects and toxicity from impaired circulation, slower absorption of medication substances and decreased muscle mass (affecting intramuscular injections)	The physical health and condition of the older person should be monitored closely and reviewed on a regular basis Assessments of injection sites should be made. Shorter needles may be needed for injections

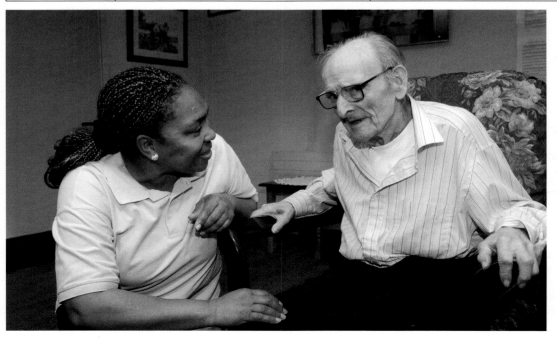

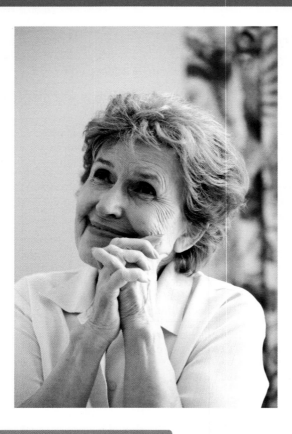

? Reflect

Individuals with dementia have rights like everybody else. In what ways do you think care workers have to work hard in protecting these individuals' rights with respect to the management of medication?

💬 Discuss

Ask your line manager or supervisor to discuss how self-medication could be promoted where you work. What are the potential challenges and how might they be overcome, if at all?

Knowledge Assessment Task

This assessment task covers HSC 3047 6.1, 6.2, 6.3.

Individuals with dementia have rights, including those relating to medication. To uphold these rights, the suitability of any medication given to individuals with dementia should be assessed as well as the means and circumstances in which the medicine is taken. Risk assessment plays an important role in promoting the individual's independence in managing medication. In this knowledge assessment task you are required to show that you know how to promote the rights of individuals when managing their medication the following.

In a format acceptable to your assessor, and providing examples from your care setting, explain the following:

1. *the importance of:*

   • *establishing consent*

   • *self-medication or active participation*

   • *dignity and privacy*

   • *confidentiality*

2. *how risk assessments can be used in promoting three individuals' independence in managing medication*

3. *how ethical issues may arise over the use of medication for individuals with dementia, giving three examples from your care setting.*

📋 Investigate

Using the internet, investigate how medication can affect individuals' dignity and privacy. What happens if individual do not consent to having medication? Is their dignity respected if everybody else thinks they should have it?

How can care workers support the use of medication?

Care workers have a key role in supporting the use of medication. In doing so they should be able to access information about an individual's medication, and demonstrate how to support an individual's use of medication in ways that promote hygiene, safety, dignity and active participation. They need to show that they can ensure medication is used or administered correctly, and also know how and when to access further information or support about the use of medication.

The safe management of medication must comply with relevant legislation and conform to local policies and agreed ways of working in the particular care setting. Following these standards and guidelines should ensure that the process of administering is safe and respectful of individuals.

Can adhering to instructions be person-centred?

It is a requirement, and good practice expected of all workers in health and social care settings, that they provide person-centred care to individuals with dementia. This includes using a person-centred approach to the appropriate and effective use of medication. Person-centredness is a way of working that aims to put the individual at the centre of the care situation, taking into account their personality, wishes and preferences.

This can be accomplished in a range of different ways, some of which are described in the case study about Milkwood on pages 158–9. A person-centred approach might include the following:

- understanding the normal routine of the individual, and accommodating the administering of medication around it

- as far as possible, meeting the preferences and wishes of the individual, for example prescribing liquids instead of tablets, having medication at a certain time (depending on the type and use of the medication) and in a preferred place (some people would rather take their medication in their room, for instance)

- helping the individual take their medication, for example giving one tablet at a time and starting with the smallest

- enabling the individual to self-administer their own medication. In social care settings this might need careful observation, and it should not be excluded or enabled without a proper risk assessment.

At all times, even when using a person-centred approach to medication management in dementia, administration instructions should be followed.

Your assessment checklist:

DEM 305

1.5 Describe how 'as required' (PRN) medication can be used to support individuals with dementia who may be in pain

2.1 Describe person-centred ways of administering medicines while adhering to administration instructions

? Reflect

Reflect on how you could get to know the normal routine of an individual with dementia. What might the challenges be?

Is all medication prescribed as a regular and consistent dose?

In some circumstances the person who is administering medication to clients or service users has some discretion about what to give. This is known as PRN medication, sometimes called 'as required' medication, because it is administered as required by the individual, but at the discretion of the person with the responsibility for giving it.

PRN stands for *pro re nata*, a Latin phrase meaning 'in the circumstances' or 'as circumstances arise'. There are a number of uses that can be made of PRN medication in dementia: to help an individual sleep at night, for instance if they are disorientated and think it is daytime; or to calm the individual if they are in extreme psychological distress following the experience of hearing voices of people who are not there.

Discuss

Discuss with a colleague the ways that individuals with dementia can be helped with taking medication. How can individuals' preferences be taken account of?

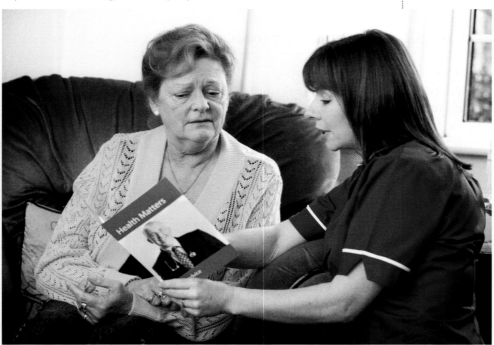

PRN medication should never be given regularly. It is for certain circumstances only. Should it appear to be needed regularly then the circumstances should be discussed with the care team, including the doctor responsible for treatment, and the care plan and prescribed medication reviewed.

However, a common use of PRN medication in dementia is for individuals who are in pain. Many older people experience pain: in their joints from arthritis or rheumatism, from skin complaints or headaches associated with eyesight problems and poor vision. Other causes of pain in older people include: poor diet and dehydration, adverse reactions to medication, and fractures.

Sometimes, individuals with dementia are not able to express themselves clearly. The care worker should therefore be vigilant for individuals in pain and take the appropriate action. This might be to:

- observe for grimacing or another indication the individual is in pain

- listen for groaning or moaning

- ask the individual if they are in pain

- be aware of changes in the way an individual walks or sits

- know about the individual's personal history, and in particular their medical history.

PRN medication for pain relief can then be offered, and any effects monitored to determine whether the pain ceases or continues. Remember that if you suspect pain you should alert and discuss it with other members of the care team and make sure the individual's care and prescription is assessed.

? Reflect

Reflect on how you communicate that you are in pain. Compare it with a person with dementia who has problems communicating.

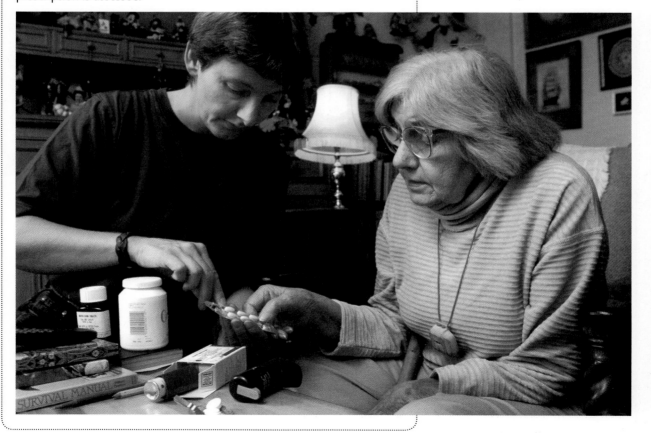

The organisation of care

The organisation of care is extremely important. Disorganised care is poor care; it is not safe and is unlikely to be effective. Medication management must be organised. The organisation of care is discussed next: accessing information about medication, supporting individuals to use medication correctly; responding to practical difficulties that might arise and looking at when and how to seek further assistance and information.

Read the following case study about Milkwood, a residential care home for older people with dementia. Isabelle, a registered nurse, is in charge; and Wandy is newly arrived from southern Africa for her first job in a UK social care setting. She is about to experience supporting the use of medication in a residential care setting for the first time.

When you have finished reading about Milkwood, answer the questions that follow.

Your assessment checklist:

DEM 305

2.2 Explain the importance of advocating for an individual with dementia who may be prescribed medication.

HSC 3047

7.1 Demonstrate how to access information about an individual's medication.

7.2 Demonstrate how to support an individual to use medication in ways that promote hygiene, safety, dignity and active participation.

7.3 Demonstrate strategies to ensure that medication is used or administered correctly.

7.4 Demonstrate how to address any practical difficulties that may arise when medication is used.

7.5 Demonstrate how and when to access further information or support about the use of medication.

Case study – Milkwood, 1: Monday

Milkwood has 30 residents, and one more is expected to be admitted later on today for assessment. The home is usually staffed by four care workers during day shifts and two at night. There is always a registered nurse on duty to lead the care team and be responsible for the daily management of Milkwood. Today Isabelle, the registered nurse, is on duty.

One of the care workers is Wandy. She is from southern Africa, and has been living in Britain for just over a month. Today she is working with two other care workers, Sophie and Benjamin.

There is a fixed routine at the home to provide structure to the day, to help residents remember what is happening and to ensure that activities including recreational and occupational activities are carried out. The morning routine begins with supporting people to get up, wash or shower, and dress before breakfast. This is soon followed by the 'medicine round', where medication is administered to residents as per their prescription chart.

After breakfast, Isabelle asks Wandy to assist her in administering medication. They both wash their hands. A trolley containing the medication is brought out to the spacious hallway where Isabelle unlocks it and sets out all the prescription cards. She asks Wandy to fetch some fresh water in a plastic jug and then starts to study the prescription charts for residents who are to have medicines.

She notes that Clarice, a 93-year-old resident, newly admitted for respite with vascular dementia, is prescribed soluble aspirin. Isabelle waits for the tablet to dissolve before taking it to Clarice while Wandy watches the trolley. Clarice says that she likes to put the aspirin in the water herself and asks if there is any reason why she shouldn't. Isabelle, who cannot think of any reason why Clarice cannot put the aspirin in to dissolve, so long as there is someone to watch her, wants to discuss it first with the care team. She also wants to conduct a risk assessment so any issues can be identified.

Bernie, one of the residents who has Alzheimer's disease, needs support to take his tablets. He finds it difficult to swallow. Isabelle notes that the tablet is 'scored', having a dividing line along its diameter. This is so that the tablet can be snapped in half. This she does, to make the two halves more manageable for Bernie. She also thinks that it would be better if he could have a liquid medicine instead, and plans to look in the BNF (British Nationals Formulary, a compendium of medicines commonly used in hospitals and other care settings to ensure medicines are used correctly and safely), to see if a liquid alternative to the tablet is available. She could then talk about the possible change with Bernie. First she discusses it with Wandy to assess whether it has been a problem for Bernie at other times.

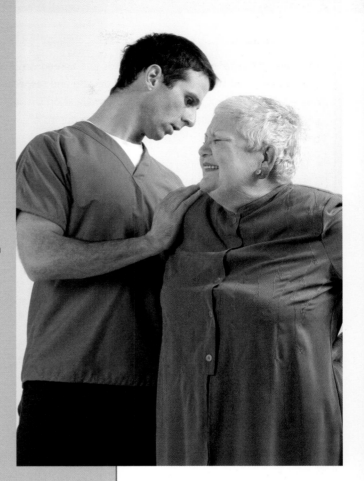

The medicine round goes as planned as the last prescription card is opened. It is for Morgan, whom Isabelle sees clearing tables. She notes that he has a cognitive enhancer, but wants to check the dose to ensure it is correct. She looks in the BNF to check as she waits for Morgan to finish clearing the tables. He then ambles to the trolley to collect his medication.

After the medicine round Isabelle talks with Wandy about Bernie's difficulty swallowing tablets. They decide to bring it up later that day at handover.

Now answer these questions.

1. How did Isabelle access information about individuals' medication?

2. In what ways did Isabelle support an individual to use medication hygienically, correctly and safely?

3. How was active participation by individuals promoted?

In the Milkwood case study, the medication round goes to plan with no hitches or unexpected difficulties. However, this is not always the case.

 Discuss

Discuss with your line manager or supervisor how medications are organised and ask to participate in medication management.

Does medication management always go to plan?

By following national and local standards and agreed ways of working, the management of medication should be safe and respectful of individuals. However, sometimes during medication management there might be some practical difficulties that arise due to organisational issues. These include:

- late delivery of medicines or delivery during busy periods such as handover times or during meals

- administering medication to a large number of clients at the same time, for example before or after a meal

- the layout of a residential facility that makes it difficult to find individuals for their medication

- distractions such as the phone ringing or an individual seeking assistance.

These are only a sample of potential practical organisational difficulties that might occur during medication management. Now read more about Milkwood.

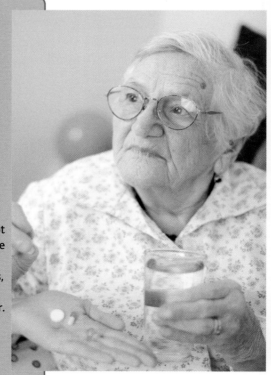

Case study – Milkwood, 2: Tuesday

Wandy is a care worker at Milkwood Residential Home for people with dementia. She is helping Isabelle, the registered nurse, to administer medication to the residents. It is now just past 1 p.m. and the residents are finishing their mid-day meal. Benjamin and Sophie are in the bathroom making sure it is clean and safe for residents' use later.

Isabelle tells her that Bernie's new medication, which has now been prescribed in liquid form because it is easier for him to swallow, has not been delivered. She asks Wandy to check the stock room for the medication box to see if it had arrived when she was unavailable. Wandy does so and returns to say it is not there.

Meanwhile Morgan has come to the trolley for his tablet, but he is not prescribed one until the evening. As Isabelle explains this to him, there is a phone call from the community chemist, wanting to speak to the person in charge. Wandy watches the trolley, which Isabelle locks, before going to the phone to ask about Bernie's medicine. It appears that the medicine is on its way but will be about another half an hour.

1. What potential practical difficulties have arisen?

2. What might Isabelle do to avoid these difficulties occurring again?

It is not easy to predict every practical difficulty that might arise in a social care setting, especially one where individuals have dementia. The individuals are vulnerable and need to be protected; abiding with standards and guidance is one way of ensuring their safety. Good day-to-day management is another way.

Isabelle might have carried out the following to ensure that potential practical difficulties were minimised:

- checked for the delivery of Bernie's new medication before she began the medicine round

- asked Wandy to tell the chemist that she would phone them back as soon as she had completed the medicine round

- arranged with the chemist and other regular callers not to phone at certain times in the future

- had all care staff on duty available at meal and medicine times.

What other practical issues might arise?

In addition to practical difficulties that arise due to organisational reasons, there are difficulties that stem from the medications themselves and failings in their management, whether the failings are due to the individual or the person responsible for administering the medication.

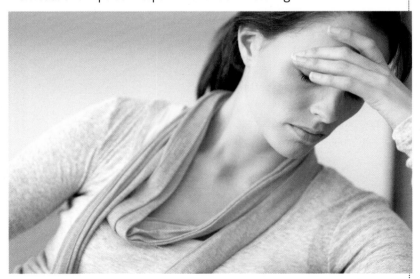

The table on the next page (figure 4.10) outlines a range of practical difficulties that might arise, and actions that can be taken in response to the difficulties.

 Investigate

Investigate the care environment where you work. To what extent does it help or hinder the organisation of medication management?

 Discuss

Discuss with colleagues what else happens when medication is administered. How far is medication administration prioritised in the daily routine of the care setting?

Figure 4.10 Practical issues surrounding medication management

Practical difficulty	What should be done
Medication might be lost, missing or damaged accidentally	In these situations the person responsible should be informed and the medication replaced as soon as practicable
An individual decides that they do not want to take medication that is prescribed for them	The purpose of the medication and potential ill-effects should be explained to the individual to establish informed consent. If the individual still does not want the medication, the prescriber and person in charge at the care setting should be informed
Difficulty in taking the medication	Some individuals with dementia lose the swallowing reflex and cannot take medication easily. Their medication might be available in alternative forms, for example as a liquid instead of tablets. The prescriber should be informed
The wrong medication is used	In these situations the individual should be observed and monitored for adverse effects, emergency action taken if necessary (consult the medication information sheet, a pharmacist or doctor or NHS Direct), and the prescriber informed
Vomiting after taking medication	The individual should be observed and monitored for a recurrence of the vomiting and any other signs of illness. The medication should not be administered again without consultation with the prescriber
Adverse reactions	These should be recorded and the individual monitored and assessed for their health status. The prescriber should be consulted
Discrepancies in records or directions for use	If there is any discrepancy in the records about what the individual should have, the medication should not be given until the correct record is established. The medication should not be given until medication, dose, time, technique and route of administration is confirmed with the prescriber

At Milkwood, Isabelle and Wandy acted as advocates for Bernie because he had difficulty swallowing tablets. It is important in social care settings that care workers act as advocates for individuals in their care who may be prescribed medication. It is even more important that they advocate for individuals with dementia because individuals might:

- be vulnerable to abuse and exploitation
- be experiencing difficulties in communication and expressing themselves
- be marginalised and not listened to
- be experiencing adverse effects or reactions that they are not aware of
- not understand the care system
- not know that options or alternative treatments might be available to them.

 Discuss

Discuss advocacy with colleagues. In what ways are they advocates for individuals in their care? What issues do they advocate on, and with whom?

What support and further information is available?

Being able to support the use of medication is an activity that is shared between different care workers and professionals, even if there is only one person who actually administers the medicine. Sometimes it is necessary to seek further information or support about the use of medication. How and when should care workers access further information or support about the use of medication? Support or further information should be sought in the following circumstances:

- *The person working with medications is not familiar with a certain medicine.* The worker should find out about any medicine that they administer. They can get more information about medication in the BNF and the medication's information leaflet. This is important. Unless the effects of and adverse reactions to a medication are understood, the caregiver will not know if it is working or if the individual is experiencing adverse effects to the medication.

- *There is a practical difficulty.* Practical difficulties can arise unexpectedly despite care workers following policies and procedures closely. Support should be sought in the first instance from the line manager or person in charge in the care setting. It is important to remember that the purpose of seeking support is not to apportion blame, but to ensure the safety of individuals and others. (Practical difficulties are discussed on pages 161–2.)

Investigate

Investigate internet sources of information about medicines. Which websites contain information that is easiest to understand? Why do you think the information they supply can be relied on, or not relied on?

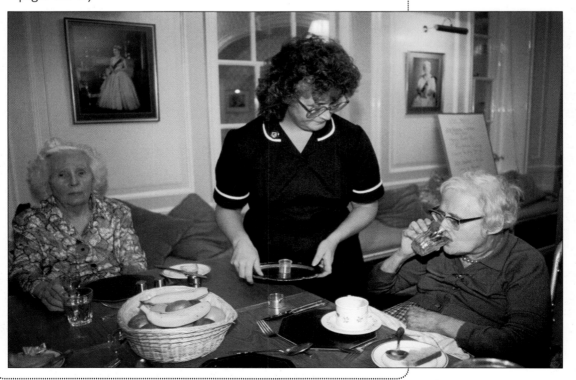

Medication management

Knowledge Assessment Task

This assessment task covers DEM 305 1.5, 2.1, 2.2.

Medication management using a person-centred approach means taking into account the wishes and preferences of the individual while complying with instructions for use of medication. For this knowledge assessment task you are required to show that you understand the appropriate use of PRN medication, person-centred ways of administering medication, and advocating for individuals with respect to their medication.

With the permission of your line manager:

1. *identify PRN medication that is prescribed in your care setting and discuss why, when and how it is used*

2. *collate this information in a format that is acceptable to your assessor*

3. *discuss your findings with your assessor*

4. *write a letter to your assessor and, in 200 words, explain the importance of advocating for one individual in your care.*

Practical Assessment Task

This assessment task covers HSC 3047 7.1, 7.2, 7.3, 7.4, 7.5.

Being able to support the use of medication is a skill that is highly valued when carried out safely and using a person-centred approach. This practical assessment task requires you to demonstrate your ability to support the use of medication, including when and how to seek further information and assistance.

With the support of your line manager and the consent of an individual in your care:

1. *access medication information about two individuals*

2. *support them in the use of medication in ways that promote hygiene, safety, dignity and active participation*

3. *support them in ways to use medication correctly*

4. *reflect on three practical difficulties that might arise, and outline to your assessor how you would address these difficulties*

5. *identify two situations when you might need to access further information and two situations when you might need to seek assistance when supporting the use of medication.*

Reflect

Reflect on the different ways that a person-centred approach to medication management is affected by dementia. Why is a person-centred approach the best option for the individual?

Discuss

Discuss with your line manager how you ensure that medication is used correctly and is administered in line with the individual's wishes and preferences. Try to discuss specific examples.

Investigate

Investigate ways to promote hygiene when administering medication. Do different techniques require different approaches to hygiene? Do they need any special measures?

Recording and reporting the use of medication

It is a requirement that workers record and report on the use of medication, including the presence of side effects and adverse reactions to medication, remembering that often individuals with dementia may not be able to report problems themselves. The use of medication and any changes to an individual associated with its use, or any other problem such as a practical difficulty, should be recorded in line with agreed ways of working.

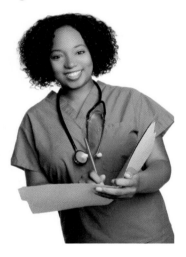

How and when a record should be made of the use of medication

Records of the use of medication should be made on the local record of administration card in line with agreed policies and ways of working:

- The record should be clear, accurate and immediate – not written sometime after the event. The record should be signed and dated, with the signature legible, so that it can be checked who administered the medicine.

- A record should be made on the record of administration card if the medication is intentionally withheld from the individual; this might be because the individual was unwell at the time, or an adverse reaction had been noted.

- A record should be made on the record of administration card if the medication is refused by the individual.

- A record should be made on the record of administration card if the individual is absent at the time, for example, when on an outing with family.

Your assessment checklist:

DEM 305

1.4 Explain the importance of recording and reporting side effects/adverse reactions to medication.

HSC 3047

8.1 Demonstrate how to record use of medication and any changes in an individual associated with it.

8.2 Demonstrate how to report on use of medication and problems associated with medication, in line with agreed ways of working.

 Discuss

Discuss with your line manager or supervisor who you should report to on the use of medication. What are the agreed ways of working when reporting on medication use?

Knowledge Assessment Task

This assessment task covers DEM 305 1.4.

Safe medication management demands proper and accurate recording and reporting. In order to understand the use of medication it is also necessary to understand any adverse reactions individuals might experience from taking medication. Any reactions must be recorded and reported to those responsible for the prescribing and management of medication. In this knowledge assessment task you are required to explain the importance of recording and reporting side effects/adverse reactions to medication.

1. *Make a list of each medication used in your care setting, and for each identify the side effects and adverse reactions using the BNF or the BNF online.*

2. *Which side effects/adverse reactions are most common for each type of medication?*

Practical Assessment Task

This assessment task covers HSC 3047 8.1, 8.2.

With the support of your line manager and the consent of individuals in your care, this practical assessment task requires you to:

1. *participate in the administering of medication to individuals*

2. *record the use of medication and any changes in an individual associated with it*

3. *report to your line manager any side effects or adverse reactions you identified*

4. *write a 200-word account about how you recorded the use of medication, who you reported to and what you reported.*

Reflect

The use of medication should always be recorded. Reflect on the potential consequences if the use of medication is not recorded.

Discuss

How are adverse reactions to medication reported? Discuss with your line manager any procedures that are in use where you work.

Investigate

Investigate how the administering of medication is recorded where you work. Are prescription administration cards used? Is reporting documented anywhere else?

Assessment checklist

The assessment of this unit is partly knowledge-based (assessing things you need to know about) and partly competence-based (assessing things you need to do in the real work environment). To complete this unit successfully, you will need to produce evidence of both your knowledge and your competence.

The knowledge-based assessment criteria for DEM 305 and HSC 3047 are listed in the 'What you need to know' table below. The practical or competence-based criteria for HSC 3047 are listed in the 'What you need to do' table opposite. Your tutor or assessor will help you to prepare for your assessment, and the tasks suggested in the chapter will help you to create the evidence you need.

Assessment criteria	What you need to know	Assessment task
DEM 305		
1.1	Outline the most common medications used to treat symptoms of dementia	Page 138
1.2	Describe how commonly-used medications affect individuals with dementia	Page 138
1.3	Explain the risks and benefits of anti-psychotic medication for individuals with dementia	Page 138
1.4	Explain the importance of recording and reporting side effects/adverse reactions to medication	Page 166
1.5	Describe how 'as required' (PRN) medication can be used to support individuals with dementia who may be in pain	Page 164
2.1	Describe person-centred ways of administering medicines while adhering to administration instructions	Page 164
2.2	Explain the importance of advocating for an individual with dementia who may be prescribed medication	Page 164

Assessment criteria	What you need to know	Assessment task
HSC 3047		
1.1	Identify legislation that governs the use of medication in social care settings	Page 134
1.2	Outline the legal classification system for medication	Page 134
1.3	Explain how and why policies and procedures or agreed ways of working must reflect and incorporate legislative requirements	Page 134
2.1	Identify common types of medication	Page 138
2.2	List conditions for which each type of medication may be prescribed	Page 138
2.3	Describe changes to an individual's physical or mental wellbeing that may indicate an adverse reaction to a medication	Page 138
3.1	Describe the roles and responsibilities of those involved in prescribing, dispensing and supporting use of medication	Page 142
3.2	Explain where responsibilities lie in relation to use of 'over the counter' remedies and supplements	Page 142
4.1	Describe the routes by which medication can be administered	Page 146
4.2	Describe different forms in which medication may be presented	Page 146
4.3	Describe materials and equipment that can assist in administering medication	Page 146
6.1	Explain the importance of the following principles in the use of medication: • consent • self-medication or active participation • dignity and privacy • confidentiality	Page 154
6.2	Explain how risk assessment can be used to promote an individual's independence in managing medication	Page 154
6.3	Describe how ethical issues that may arise over the use of medication can be addressed	Page 154

Assessment criteria	What you need to do	Assessment task
HSC 3047		
5.1	Demonstrate how to receive supplies of medication in line with agreed ways of working	Page 149
5.2	Demonstrate how to store medication safely	Page 149
5.3	Demonstrate how to dispose of unused or unwanted medication safely	Page 149
7.1	Demonstrate how to access information about an individual's medication	Page 164
7.2	Demonstrate how to support an individual to use medication in ways that promote hygiene, safety, dignity and active participation	Page 164
7.3	Demonstrate strategies to ensure that medication is used or administered correctly	Page 164
7.4	Demonstrate how to address any practical difficulties that may arise when medication is used	Page 164
7.5	Demonstrate how and when to access further information or support about the use of medication	Page 164
8.1	Demonstrate how to record use of medication and any changes in an individual associated with it	Page 166
8.2	Demonstrate how to report on use of medication and problems associated with medication, in line with agreed ways of working	Page 166

5 | The nutritional requirements of individuals with dementia

DEM 302
LO1 Understand the nutritional needs that are unique to individuals with dementia

- ▶ Describe how cognitive, functional and emotional changes associated with dementia can affect eating, drinking and nutrition

- ▶ Explain how poor nutrition can contribute to an individual's experience of dementia

- ▶ Outline how other health and emotional conditions may affect the nutritional needs of an individual with dementia

- ▶ Explain the importance of recognising and meeting an individual's personal and cultural preferences for food and drink

- ▶ Explain why it is important to include a variety of food and drink in the diet of an individual with dementia

DEM 302
LO2 Understand the effect that mealtime environments can have on an individual with dementia

- ▶ Describe how mealtime cultures and environments can be a barrier to meeting the nutritional needs of an individual with dementia

- ▶ Describe how mealtime environments and food presentation can be designed to help an individual to eat and drink

- ▶ Describe how a person-centred approach can support an individual, with dementia at different levels of ability, to eat and drink

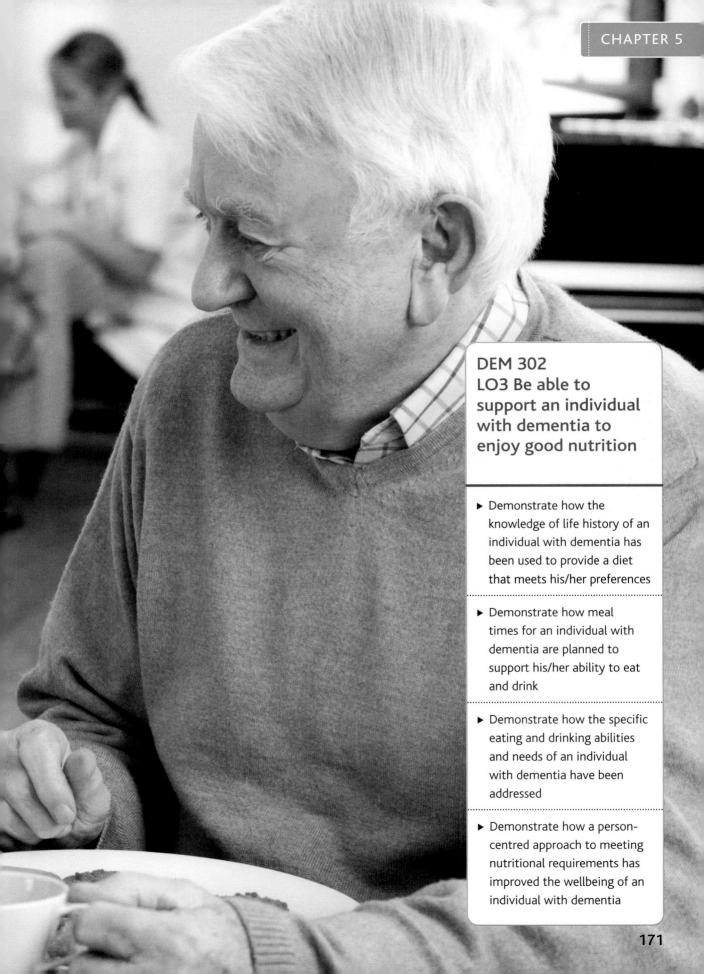

CHAPTER 5

**DEM 302
LO3 Be able to support an individual with dementia to enjoy good nutrition**

▶ Demonstrate how the knowledge of life history of an individual with dementia has been used to provide a diet that meets his/her preferences

▶ Demonstrate how meal times for an individual with dementia are planned to support his/her ability to eat and drink

▶ Demonstrate how the specific eating and drinking abilities and needs of an individual with dementia have been addressed

▶ Demonstrate how a person-centred approach to meeting nutritional requirements has improved the wellbeing of an individual with dementia

Nutritional needs unique to individuals with dementia

Introduction to this chapter

This chapter covers the learning and assessment requirements of DEM 302 *Understand and meet the nutritional requirements of individuals with dementia*. The chapter focuses on the ways in which dementia can affect the nutritional status of individuals, as well as the impact of nutrition on a person's experience of dementia. It will help you understand the need to create environments that encourage healthy eating and drinking and guide you in using a range of person-centred skills to enable individuals with dementia to eat and drink well.

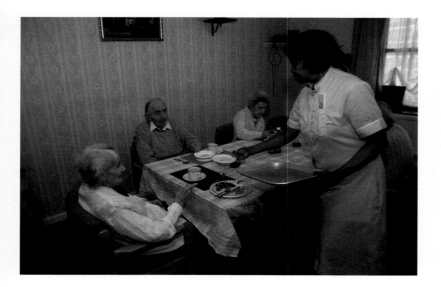

Your assessment criteria:

DEM 302

1.1 Describe how cognitive, functional and emotional changes associated with dementia can affect eating, drinking and nutrition.

🔑 Key terms

Cognitive: mental processes to do with thinking, awareness, knowledge, perception, reasoning and judgment

Delusional ideas: fixed beliefs or perceptions that persist despite evidence to the contrary

Functional: able to fulfil everyday functions and carry out usual behaviours

Nutritional status: physical health in relation to the consumption of nutrients

Paranoia: an unfounded or exaggerated negative state of distrust towards objects and/or people, which can form part of a delusion

In what ways can dementia affect nutrition?

Dementia does not cause weight loss, but it does affect the way a person thinks, behaves and feels, so that everyday activities such as eating and drinking can be detrimentally affected. Over time, this can impact on a person's **nutritional status** and his or her health and wellbeing. As a health and social care worker it is vital to recognise the challenges a person with dementia faces in eating a healthy and balanced diet, because of the impact of:

- cognitive changes
- functional changes
- emotional changes.

❓ Reflect

Think about your diet, the foods you eat and what you drink. Consider how day-to-day changes, such as feeling upset, having a cold, or being anxious, impact on your eating patterns. Try to relate this to the fluctuations in appetite that a person with dementia might experience.

Look at the table in Figure 5.1, which shows the main changes associated with dementia that impact on nutrition. Remember that not all individuals with dementia will experience all of these changes, but it is likely that most will experience some.

 Discuss

Talk with colleagues about your experiences with individuals whose cognitive, functional and emotional deficits from dementia impact on their nutrition. Share strategies for managing these difficulties.

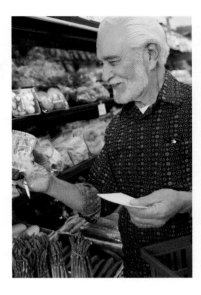

Figure 5.1 How dementia impacts on nutrition

Impacts of dementia on nutrition		
Cognitive **changes**	Functional **changes**	**Emotional changes**
Confusion and disorientation may mean a person no longer responds to hunger and thirst, so he or she may forget to eat, try to eat non-food items, or not recognise cues for eating, such as a place setting at table, or plate of food **Memory difficulties** interfere with shopping for, preparing and cooking food; keeping to normal mealtime routines; and remembering whether food has been eaten, so that meals may be skipped or eaten more often, and dietary variety diminishes **Concentration difficulties** make it hard to remain focused on tasks connected with shopping, food preparation, cooking, eating and drinking	**Visio-spatial perception changes** interfere with recognising or using cutlery and crockery, and bringing food and drink to the mouth effectively **Sensory perceptions** mean taste can be dulled or changed, interfering with appetite **Oral and dental difficulties** may result in reduced saliva production, problems in chewing to soften food, plus a weakened swallowing reflex, increasing the risk of choking and inhaling food into the lungs, where it can cause pneumonia **Challenging behaviours** caused by damage from dementia to specific areas of the brain can result in hoarding food, sexual disinhibition, restlessness, or anger outbursts at meal times, as well as eating food from others' plates and smearing food **Communication issues** can make it difficult for a person to understand nutritional needs and have preferences understood **Reduced or increased digestive activity** can cause bowel changes, such as constipation or diarrhoea, as well as gastric reflux and indigestion, which make a person less likely to eat **Medication** can cause drowsiness, lack of sensation, taste and other side-effects connected with digestion	**Anxiety** is a common feature of dementia and meal times can increase stress levels, especially if a person feels under pressure to eat, is frightened of choking, or is confused by the surroundings and others' expectations **Agitation** may mean a person cannot sit still and focus on eating, leading to fiddling with the meal setting, getting up and pacing **Depression** commonly accompanies dementia and tends to be under-diagnosed, leading to increasing withdrawal and isolation and reduced appetite **Low motivation** due to depression may lead to inability to manage simple tasks such as providing food and drink for oneself Paranoia **and** delusions can be a feature of dementia and might impact on nutrition if a person believes food is being tampered with or he/she is not worthy to eat it, for example

How does poor nutrition affect people with dementia?

Malnutrition occurs when insufficient foods, or foods with poor nutritional value, are eaten. Dehydration is also a common feature of malnutrition, where insufficient fluid is drunk through the day. The key issues caused by poor nutrition are:

- disruption to body systems

- vulnerability to illness and disease.

Disruption to body systems

Food and fluids are essential to the normal functioning of body systems, and a regular intake of a healthy range of food and drinks (see page 183) is necessary to avoid damage and disease. The symptoms of such damage will all be harder for a person with dementia to manage. Dehydration causes symptoms such as a dry mouth, nausea, reduced appetite and electrolyte imbalance. This imbalance in turn causes cardiac irregularities and confusion, in addition to the confusion already present from dementia. Without adequate fluid throughout the day, kidney function is reduced, increasing the risk of urinary infections and incontinence. The skin, too, is affected by dehydration. Combined with difficulties managing personal hygiene because of dementia, this can mean that skin becomes sore and could break down.

Vulnerability to illness

A person whose body systems are damaged by malnutrition and dehydration is more vulnerable to infection and less able to fight it. Someone who is ill has a reduced appetite, will be less active, less mobile and has an increased likelihood of further complications. Symptoms of dementia will be magnified and it will be harder to manage the tasks of everyday life. Look at Figure 5.2 opposite, which identifies the negative effects of malnutrition and dehydration.

Key terms

Dehydration: the loss of water and salts essential for normal body function

Electrolyte imbalance: disruption to the levels of essential salts in the body, which impact on body function and can lead to death

Malnutrition: deficiency of nutrients due to inadequate or imbalanced diet, interfering with healthy functioning of the body

Investigate

The Patients Association (www.patients-association.com) produced a leaflet in 2011 entitled 'Malnutrition – how to spot the signs and what to expect from treatment'. Use work, library or internet sources to read through the information and consider how it relates to the individuals you care for.

Cardiovascular and circulatory system:
affecting heart, blood vessels and circulation causing cardiac irregularities; poor healing; fragile skin

Digestive system:
affecting the processing of food causing diarrhoea/constipation; electrolyte imbalance; weight loss/weight gain; causing mouth/dental soreness; vitamin and mineral deficiency; anaemia

Urinary system:
affecting excretion through kidneys and bladder causing infections; incontinence

Malnutrition and dehydration

Nervous system:
affecting senses and cognition causing memory loss; confusion; wandering

Muscular-skeletal system:
affecting bones, muscles and movement causing muscle weakness; reduced mobility; falls

Respiratory system:
affecting breathing causing shallow breathing, increasing susceptibility to infection

Endocrine system:
affecting hormone control and dealing with stress causing body temperature imbalance; anxiety

Figure 5.2 Negative effects of malnutrition and dehydration

Case study

Vita has not been eating well since his wife died. He receives a meals service each day, but often forgets to eat his food. Family members notice he has lost weight, and when he falls and breaks his wrist, hospital staff diagnose dehydration as well. Vita finds it hard to cope in the strange surroundings of the ward and calls for his wife constantly.

1. How might a lack of nutrition have increased Vita's vulnerability to falling?

2. How might dementia complicate Vita's health and affect his ability to recover in hospital?

3. If you were caring for Vita, what would you suggest to improve his nutritional status?

? | Reflect

The Equality and Human Rights Commission report of November 2011 investigated the home care system in England. It highlighted cases where people unable to feed themselves were given no help and their meals went uneaten. Think about why this might happen in care environments.

 Discuss

Share with colleagues what you have noticed about people with dementia who have lost significant weight. Generate some ideas for increasing their calorific intake and improving the nutritional value of meals throughout the day.

How can health and emotional conditions affect nutrition for a person with dementia?

For many older people it is likely that dementia is just one element of a complex health and welfare picture. A common effect of ageing is wear and tear on the body, which can result in increasing illness, disease and disability. Along with physical effects come emotional ones, such as anxiety, frustration, anger, fear about the future and sadness. Think about the impact on nutrition of:

- medical conditions

- health issues

- moods and emotions.

Key terms

Hyperglycaemia: abnormally high blood sugar

Hypoglycaemia: abnormally low blood sugar

Reflect

Think about how your different moods affect your appetite and influence what you eat.

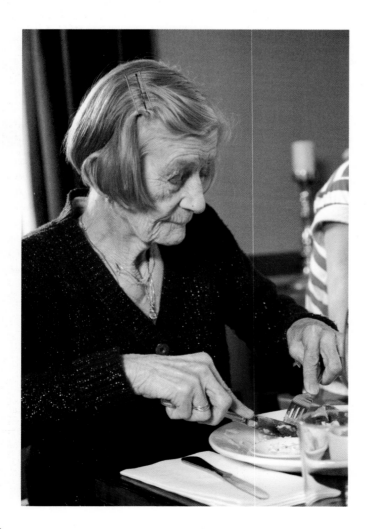

Discuss

Talk with colleagues about individuals you care for who have medical conditions as well as dementia. Consider the ways that the symptoms complicate the person's dementia.

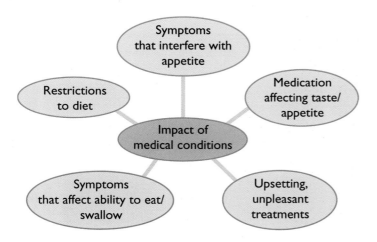

An example of a medical condition affecting nutrition and impacting on dementia is diabetes, where diet must be balanced alongside tablets or insulin injections. People with dementia may forget about dietary restrictions and whether medication has been taken. Symptoms of unstable diabetes, such as **hyper-** or **hypo-glycaemia**, may be mistaken for confusion associated with dementia, and go untreated. Consider also the impact of medical conditions such as a stroke, Parkinson's disease and rheumatoid arthritis.

Figure 5.3 The impact of medical conditions on nutrition

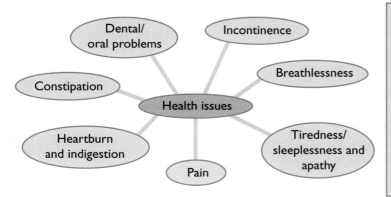

As a person ages, body systems no longer work so efficiently, and the symptoms of this are harder for a person with dementia to recognise, make sense of, communicate and manage. This may have an impact on nutrition. For example, pain may mean a person can't get comfortable to eat, or missing teeth might make it difficult to chew food. Even in hospital or care environments, health issues for people with dementia can go unnoticed.

Figure 5.4 Health issues affecting nutrition

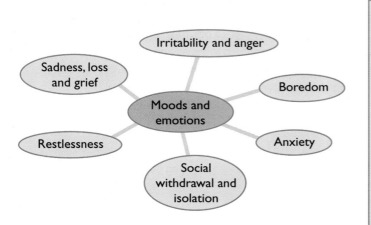

Dementia does not mean people no longer feel emotions, some of which can interfere with wanting to eat and drink. It can be harder for a person with dementia to manage the emotional effects of ageing and know how to seek support. People with insight into their memory loss may avoid friends and family out of embarrassment, and consequent social isolation can reduce dietary intake. A person can become apathetic without stimulus, and is less likely to eat. Anxiety makes it hard for a person to concentrate on food and increases restlessness, which burns more calories, leading to weight loss.

Figure 5.5 Mental health and emotional difficulties affecting nutrition

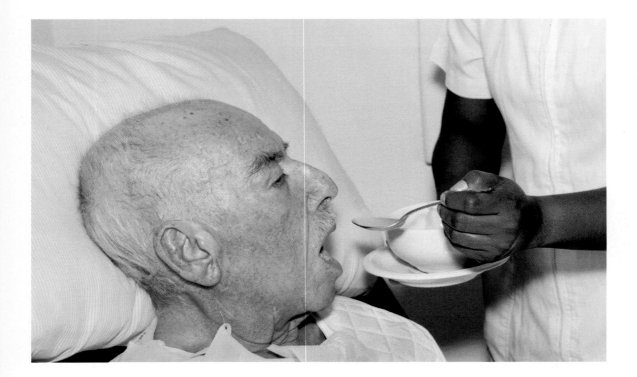

Case study

Sybil has a history of constipation, which is much harder for her to manage now she has dementia and this increases her anxiety. She can never remember if she has passed a motion, so spends a long time straining on the toilet, which has resulted in haemorrhoids (piles). She decides to eat less to reduce the need to go to the toilet, but is becoming more apathetic and less active as a result. Sybil's GP, district nurses and home care team meet to discuss how they can help Sybil.

1. In what ways has dementia impacted on Sybil's ability to manage her constipation?

2. What could be said to Sybil to explain why eating less is not a good solution?

3. Which foods would help Sybil to keep her digestion working well?

 Discuss

Talk together with colleagues about different methods and approaches you use to try to encourage an older person with dementia to eat.

 Investigate

Using library, internet and work sources, find out what you can about dietary fibre, why it is needed and the foods that contain it. You could create a poster of your findings to display at work.

Knowledge Assessment Task

This assessment task covers DEM 302 1.1, 1.2, 1.3.

Dementia impacts on what a person eats and drinks, commonly leading to a poorer nutritional intake. Reduced nutrition has a negative effect on a person's experience of dementia.

To complete this task you need to read each statement in the chart opposite carefully, explain possible reasons for the situation and provide suggestions for managing it.

1. Ellen believes the food in the care home has been tampered with and refuses to eat her meals.

Reason:

Management:

2. Vince finds it harder to concentrate and focus and no longer manages to shop and cook, but his neighbour doesn't mind bringing him small items such as bread and milk, so he mostly eats sandwiches now.

Reason:

Management:

3. Biddy stopped going to the lunch club because she finds it embarrassing when she can't remember people's names, and it doesn't seem worth bothering with a midday meal any more.

Reason:

Management:

4. Derek keeps choking when he's eating, which makes him anxious around meal times.

Reason:

Management:

5. Winston frequently removes his dentures, wraps them in tissues and hides them away, forgetting where he has put them.

Reason:

Management:

Keep the written work that you produce as evidence for your assessment.

> **? Reflect**
>
> *Imagine you lived in a care home. Think about how it would feel to be convinced that someone is against you and might be trying to inflict harm on you in a way that isn't obvious to others. How would this make you feel about eating meals that are cooked by a person you don't know, with foods that you have not shopped for or prepared yourself, in a kitchen you have never seen?*

Why is it important to acknowledge personal and cultural food and drink preferences?

Your assessment criteria:

DEM 302

1.4 Explain the importance of recognising and meeting an individual's personal and cultural preferences for food and drink.

The need to eat and drink is shared by everyone, but the way meals are prepared, the different food types and ways of eating are influenced by a person's background and likes and dislikes. Personal and cultural preferences take on greater significance for a person with dementia, because they help to trigger memories and provide a familiar structure and routine. This gives each person a sense of unique individuality. Factors to consider are set out in the table below.

Figure 5.6 Cultural and personal food and drink preferences

Term	Preference	Example
Ethnicity	Foods usual to a country/region; food prepared and eaten according to custom	Agnes is Scottish and has had porridge with salt and no sugar or milk for breakfast since she was a child
Religion	Prohibited foods; specific preparation of foods; particular food for religious occasions	A Kosher diet is given to Ben, who is Jewish: meat is prepared according to custom and certain foods are included or excluded
Beliefs	Vegetarian, vegan	Marnie is given rissoles made with lentils as a vegetarian alternative to meat
Culture/ background	Social and family routines; celebration meals (these link to the power of reminiscence to whet appetites)	Because Rick's family used to eat tea in front of the television on Sundays, the care home arrange for his wife to continue this practice and he always eats really well
Individual taste	Likes and dislikes	Fish was never a favourite of Pete's, even though he was a fisherman for 30 years

The importance of meeting dietary preferences

The main reason for finding out about food preferences is that people are more likely to eat and drink well if they are enjoying their meal, but there are additional benefits as well. These are set out in the diagram opposite (figure 5.7).

Key terms

Culture: beliefs and ways of behaving that are characteristic of a particular social, ethnic, or age group

Institutionalisation: the process of conforming to the routines and usual behaviours expected within an institution and suppressing individuality

Discuss

Talk with colleagues about routines to do with meal times that take place where you work. Discuss whether these have the potential to ignore the personal preferences of individuals.

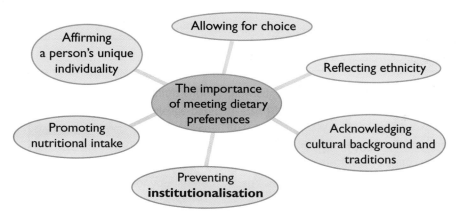

Figure 5.7 Reasons for meeting dietary preferences

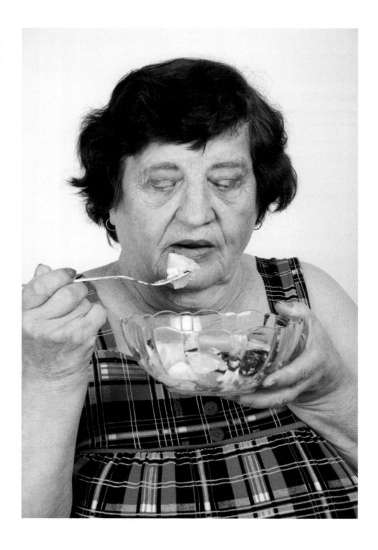

 Investigate

Using internet and library sources, find out about traditions related to food from different countries. Consider such matters as communal eating with fingers out of a shared bowl; use of chopsticks; rituals related to religious festivals.

? **Reflect**

Think about traditions and rituals associated with food that took place when you were a child.

Finding out about the preferences of a person with dementia

A person with dementia may have difficulty identifying preferences and communicating these verbally. It is important for care workers to encourage a person with dementia to express his or her wishes and notice the meals that appear to be enjoyed. Speak also with family about their relative's likes and dislikes, recording the information for all staff members including the person doing the cooking. Be specific. For example, if a person likes fish, find out which meals containing fish are preferred. Also, check whether individuals want to try something new, because tastes can change and sometimes the dulling of taste and smell associated with dementia can mean a person needs more strongly flavoured, highly seasoned food.

Your assessment criteria:

DEM 302

1.5 Explain why it is important to include a variety of food and drink in the diet of an individual with dementia.

Investigate

Using library, Internet and work sources, find out more about vitamins, such as vitamins A, B12, C and D, and how these contribute to the functioning of the body. Find out which foods contain these vitamins and make a table to illustrate your findings.

Case study

Bettina is from Portugal, and as her dementia progresses she stops speaking English and reverts to Portuguese. All day she paces the corridors of the care home, where staff constantly try to persuade her to sit down. She doesn't usually settle, even to eat or drink, until late evening, long after the last meal has been served. The manager is concerned because at the monthly weight check Bettina has lost 2 kg.

1. How can staff reflect something of Bettina's cultural background in the care they offer around food and meal times?

2. How might staff increase Bettina's nutritional intake?

3. What observations should staff be making to monitor the situation?

Why is it important to provide nutritional variety?

Most people prefer to eat a varied diet, but variety is also necessary to provide a range of nutritional elements that are contained in different food types and required for healthy functioning. Consider:

• balanced menu choice

• stimulating appetite

• food combinations for optimum nutrition

• food fortification and supplements.

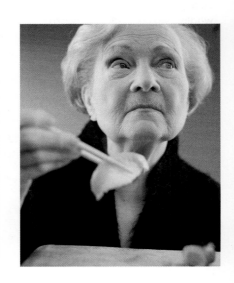

Providing a balanced menu

People need a balance of different nutrients in their diet. The range of these is illustrated in the diagram below (figure 5.8). If you help a person with dementia to shop and cook, you need to balance nutritional advice about what to buy alongside food preferences. For example, a person may not like (or be unable to chew) vegetables or fruit, which would reduce the intake of vitamins, minerals and fibre. But the person may be happy to eat these puréed to form soup or pulped in a smoothie.

In care environments, spend time helping a person select items from the menu, bearing in mind that something chosen in advance may not be remembered when the meal arrives. It may help to write choices on a calendar, or use pictures of meals as a memory and communication aid.

Reflect

Think about foods that might be good to tempt a person's appetite after they have been unwell or when they're feeling upset.

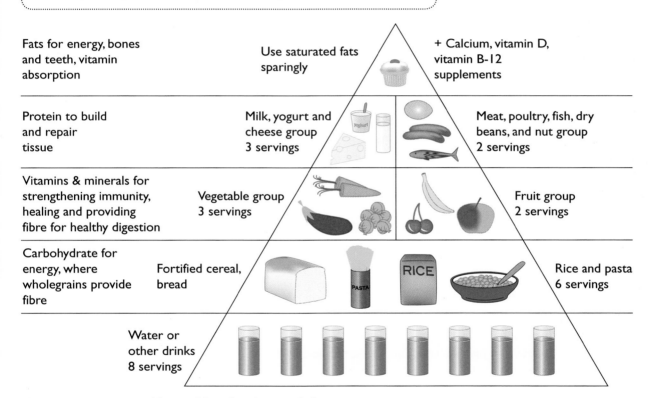

Fats for energy, bones and teeth, vitamin absorption

Use saturated fats sparingly

+ Calcium, vitamin D, vitamin B-12 supplements

Protein to build and repair tissue

Milk, yogurt and cheese group
3 servings

Meat, poultry, fish, dry beans, and nut group
2 servings

Vitamins & minerals for strengthening immunity, healing and providing fibre for healthy digestion

Vegetable group
3 servings

Fruit group
2 servings

Carbohydrate for energy, where wholegrains provide fibre

Fortified cereal, bread

RICE

Rice and pasta
6 servings

Water or other drinks
8 servings

Figure 5.8 How to provide nutritional variety each day. Remember that some foods contain combined nutritional value, such as cheese, which is fat and protein

 Discuss

Talk together with colleagues about designing menu plans that include balanced and nutritious meals suitable for an older person with dementia.

Stimulating appetite

If a meal is enjoyable it is more likely to be eaten. Stimulating the senses increases appetite, so consider delicious aromas, interesting textures, the sizzle of something frying and the sight of steam wafting from saucepans, all of which increase anticipation. Helping a person pour a drink from a jug involves touch and the sound of liquid pouring or ice cubes chinking, which can stimulate a person to drink. Flavouring water with cordial makes it more palatable for some. It may be appropriate to offer an alcoholic drink such as a Sherry before meals, but check whether this is desired and compatible with medication. Using a toaster is a simple way in which people can benefit from seeing and smelling food in preparation. Brief and gentle exercise before meal times also increases appetite and makes a person feel ready to eat.

Optimising nutrition

The benefits of nutrition are increased by making sure food is not overcooked, which destroys vitamin content. On the other hand some foods should be avoided with older people, such as raw or underdone eggs, because these can cause food poisoning, which can have a devastating effect on nutritional status. Figure 5.8 provides guidelines on recommended servings of different food groups to provide optimum nutrition, although be aware that less active people need less carbohydrate. Eight glasses of fluid per day (unless restricted due to another medical condition, such as congestive heart failure) are recommended, but can include drinks other than water.

Food fortification and supplements

Sometimes it is not possible for a person with dementia to take in adequate nutrition in meals alone, and it may be necessary to use supplementary feeding to fortify the diet. Supplements come in different forms, illustrated in figure 5.9 opposite. These should only be used after consultation with a doctor or dietician/nutritionist. Be aware that as a carer you may be the first person to recognise that a person is not eating or drinking well, and it is your responsibility to bring it to the attention of your manager, who can refer the person to a specialist practitioner (see page 190).

Key term

Supplementary feeding: programme in which food is provided to individuals specifically to prevent or treat malnutrition

Investigate

Using library, internet and work sources, find out more about vitamins, such as vitamins A, B12, C and D, and how these contribute to the functioning of the body. Find out which foods contain these vitamins and make a table to illustrate your findings.

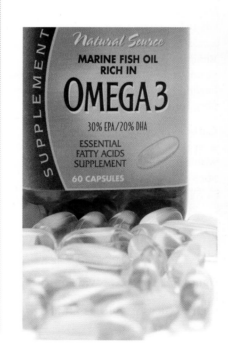

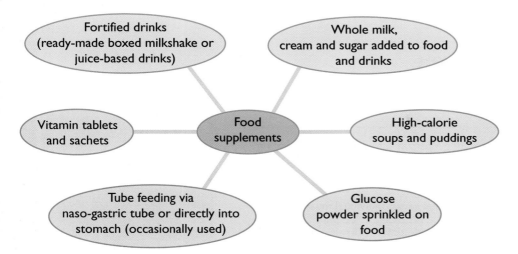

Figure 5.9 Methods of fortifying diet

Knowledge Assessment Task

This assessment task covers DEM 302 1.4, 1.5.

Meals provided for older people with dementia need to reflect a person's cultural and personal preferences while also providing a varied and nutritionally balanced diet. Design a whole day's menu including drinks and breakfast, lunch, dinner, morning and afternoon snack for the following individuals, explaining your choices.

1. *Bert has traditional tastes, enjoying old-fashioned food from his childhood. He is the son of a dairy farmer and says his mother cooked plain food and made lovely pastry and cakes. Luckily Bert is not overweight, and as he walks a lot he has a hearty appetite.*

2. *Mrs Patel has been off her food since she had flu. She has lost weight and will only tolerate small amounts of food through the day, sometimes wanting only a drink or snack rather than a full meal. Her family say she prefers eating traditional meals from southern India and does not really like Western food.*

3. *Lexi is always ready for her breakfast and eats well at this time of day, but staff at the care home find it hard to persuade her to sit and eat for other meals, and often leave finger food for her to take as she passes.*

Keep the written work that you produce as evidence for your assessment.

 Investigate

Using internet, local community and work sources, find out about the provision of meal services at home in your area and the ways they ensure nutritional value, balance and variety.

 Reflect

Think about going out to restaurants and favourite dishes you enjoy. Identify the elements of the food and service that add to your enjoyment. Consider whether you could incorporate some of these touches where you work.

 Discuss

Talk with colleagues about the menu choice provided to the individuals you care for. Consider the nutritional variety and balance, and suggest ways to enhance this.

Effects of mealtime environments on individuals with dementia

In what ways can meal times create barriers to healthy eating?

Meal times can be a barrier preventing a person with dementia from eating a healthy diet, whether at home or in a communal environment. Look at the table (figure 5.10) below, which highlights how this can happen.

Figure 5.10 Negative aspects of communal versus individual meal times

Communal meal times	Individual meal times
Can be noisy and distracting if a person with dementia is easily over-stimulated and unable to concentrate on eating a meal with others	People with dementia can become isolated and may not bother to shop, cook or eat regularly; appetite may decrease; there may be a lack of nutritional variety; poor food hygiene may lead to food poisoning
It can be stressful for a person with dementia to meet the social expectations of others, such as acceptable manners and following conversations	Lone individuals with dementia cannot observe and follow the example of others eating around the table
The rigidity of a meal eaten together at a specific time does not allow for a person with dementia to eat when they please or when they feel hungry	There are no prompts such as a dining table laid ready for a meal with place settings, flowers or other decorations, especially when celebrating events such as birthdays
It can be embarrassing for a person who needs aids to eat food and who may drop food or dribble	There is no stimulus to appetite such as seeing meals set down on the table and witnessing others enjoying their food
Some people with dementia need to 'graze' – that is, eat small amounts of food while moving around, or getting up and down during a meal	Without prompts, meals provided by a meal delivery service may be forgotten or unfinished

Your assessment criteria:

DEM 302

2.1 Describe how mealtime cultures and environments can be a barrier to meeting the nutritional needs of an individual with dementia.

2.2 Describe how mealtime environments and food presentation can be designed to help an individual to eat and drink.

Investigate

Ask your manager if you can experiment with playing different types of music during meal times to see whether certain music, or radio stations, or no music, encourages eating.

Case study

Bridie was a sociable person before her stroke, which resulted in vascular dementia. She is embarrassed by the need to feed herself with a spoon and that she drops food. She also dribbles and has a weakened swallowing reflex. Although Bridie asks to have her meals in her room, staff prefer her to eat at a communal dining table where they can help her quickly if she chokes.

1. What would you do to reconcile the conflicting wishes of staff and resident in this situation?
2. What are your reasons for these decisions?
3. How would you arrange the dining environment to meet Bridie's needs more effectively?

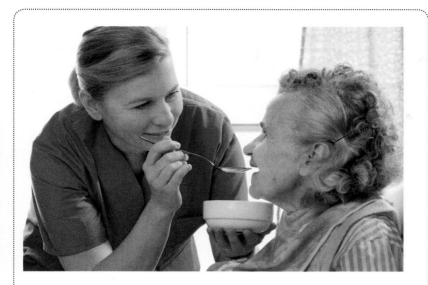

? Reflect

Think about different environments where you enjoy eating meals, perhaps outdoor picnics or breakfast in bed, and consider whether these ideas might work for those you care for.

💬 Discuss

Talk with colleagues about the various aids you use when helping people with dementia to eat, and share what you have found most useful for particular individuals and circumstances.

How can the environment and food presentation encourage eating and drinking?

There are positive steps you can take to improve the intake of food and drink for individuals with dementia. Consider:

- conducive mealtime environments

- food presentation.

Conducive mealtime environments

The surroundings for eating can be as important as the food that is provided. Be flexible in your thinking, and remember that individuals with dementia may wish to eat some meals at the dining table and others in bed, or from a tray on their lap. Some may eat standing up, or while moving. Also be flexible with timings, because set meal times may no longer have meaning for people with dementia, who might wish to eat when they feel like it or when they are hungry.

Be sensitive when you are seating groups of people together. Allow for choice of company to be expressed and make sure individuals and their specific needs are compatible with each other. For example, don't sit two restless people together or they will be easily distracted. It can help to have staff members eating a meal alongside individuals with dementia, their example providing prompts about using cutlery and drinking and eating well. People will eat more successfully if they feel relaxed and stress free.

Think about the physical surroundings in a dining area. Make sure it is warm and light. Provide information, such as signs that state it is a dining area, perhaps with a clock-face to show the time of the next meal. A menu (preferably illustrated) provides a prompt and helps to prepare a person for eating a meal. Items related to eating also nudge the memory, such as crockery displayed on a dresser, tablecloths and napkins. Show thoughtfulness by displaying flowers or candles, out of reach of those who may harm themselves. Look at figure 5.11 to remind yourself of each factor to consider.

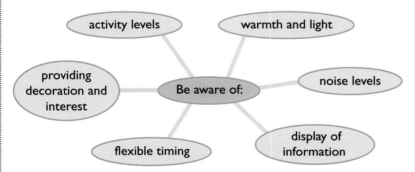

Figure 5.11 Creating conducive mealtime environments

Range of food presentations

The way that food is presented impacts on eating, and an attractive-looking plate can stimulate appetite. A huge portion of food can be off-putting, whereas a smaller portion, presented carefully, looks appetising. A garnish of salad, fruit or herbs is an attractive finish that shows attention to detail. As well as presenting a meal attractively, always provide appropriate sauces and seasoning.

According to the needs of a person with dementia, some meals need to be presented differently to enable an individual to eat safely. Look at the diagram (figure 5.12 opposite).

- A soft diet shouldn't require chewing, and includes foods that can be eaten with a fork or spoon alone, such as mashed potatoes.

- Puréed food is required by someone with a weak swallowing reflex. Always liquidise different food types separately to preserve their original colour, making sure you let the person know what the meal consists of, because this may not be obvious.

- The consistency of drinks and some foods, such as soup and puddings, may need to be thickened to provide bulk for someone who is likely to choke.

? | Reflect

Consider how it might feel to have to eat a soft diet or even puréed food. What do you think might become more important to you as a result of this restriction?

- Chopping food may help a person with dementia to eat independently, but do this in the kitchen to avoid embarrassment.

- Finger foods such as sandwiches and bite-size items can be eaten without cutlery. This is an advantage for people whose cognitive and functional skills are affected, but who wish to eat independently without drawing attention to their difficulty.

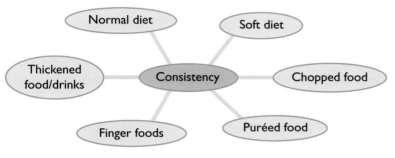

Figure 5.12 Food and drink consistencies

Discuss

Talk together with colleagues about ways to ensure that a person with dementia who is restless can still manage to eat enough calories to prevent weight loss.

Case study

The manager of The Pines care home wants to create a reminiscence dining area. The average age of the residents means they mostly grew up and had their families in the 1940s and 1950s.

1. What do you think might be the reasons for the manager's decision?

2. What sort of items do you think might fit in a 1940s and 1950s reminiscence dining room?

3. What ideas about dining room design do you have to encourage people with dementia to eat?

 Investigate

Using library and internet sources, gather together information about indoor and outdoor plants that can be grown in pots and bear fruit that can be eaten, such as tomatoes, cress and lettuces. These types of plants can be tended and eaten by residents in a care home or at a day centre.

How does a person-centred approach support different levels of ability to eat and drink?

It is a mistake to think all people with dementia require the same support to eat and drink. Everyone is different. You will need to consider:

- individualised assistance to eat and drink

- providing appropriate aids.

Individualised assistance to eat and drink

Your role is to find ways to enable individuals to eat a healthy balanced diet. You need to get to know each unique person and build a trusting relationship with them. Family members can often provide insights too. Assistance from the following specialist practitioners may be available:

- dietician – to tailor diet

- speech and language specialist – to manage oral and swallowing difficulties

- occupational therapist – to advise on aids

- physiotherapist – to advise on posture and positioning

- dentist – to ensure teeth and gums are disease free and dentures fit.

Make sure you follow instructions from specialists and record progress.

It is bad practice to encourage a person to fit into a routine that suits the service provider – the service must be tailored to the individual. There is also no point in insisting a person sits at a table and eats, whether with others or alone, if he or she does not wish to do so, and it is never acceptable to force-feed a person.

Providing aids appropriate to the individual

No single aid for eating and drinking will suit every individual with dementia, even when they have similar physical difficulties. For example, one person who has problems drinking from a cup because it is difficult to control the flow of fluid and tends to choke may find using a straw helps, whereas another likes to spoon the drink to the mouth, while another manages better with a beaker that has a spout. As a care worker you must explore the different possibilities along with each person to find what suits his or her needs and preferences, and be aware that choices might change over time.

Your assessment criteria:

DEM 302

2.3 Describe how a person-centred approach can support an individual, with dementia at different levels of ability, to eat and drink.

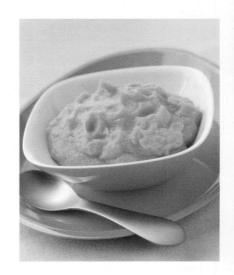

Cognitive changes make it difficult for some people to differentiate between the table and the plate. A contrasting coloured tablecloth, or a coloured rim around crockery, can help. Sometimes plastic cutlery is preferred to metal, a fork to a spoon, or a teaspoon to a dessert spoon. Your job is to find out and share your findings so that care can be tailored to the person, regardless of who provides the care. Look at the table (figure 5.13) for the best ways to help a person with dementia to eat and drink, as well as what to avoid.

Figure 5.13 Helping a person with dementia to eat and drink

Dos and Don'ts of assisting a person with dementia at meal times	
DO ✓	DON'T ✗
Work out (preferably with the person) how much help is needed	Don't intervene and take over to feed a person to save time, or mess
Ensure each person is supported in the chair or bed, not in pain, doesn't need the toilet, and is given an opportunity to wash hands	Don't rush the person or give the impression you don't have time
Ensure suitable eating aids and protection for clothes are provided	Don't share aids between people during meals, or refer to napkins as 'bibs'
Prepare a place setting with appropriate cutlery, crockery, seasoning, sauces and a drink	Do not carry plates of food around without a tray
Sit at the same level, or lower than the person you are helping to eat and at an angle, not side by side	Never stand over a person when assisting with eating
Focus your attention on the person, making sure he or she can hear and see you	Do not have conversations with staff members when helping a person; do not assist more than one person to eat at a time
Check the temperature of food in the kitchen before serving by taking a teaspoonful and putting it on your inner wrist	Do not serve microwaved food without stirring and leaving to stand; do not dip your finger in food to check temperature
Combine different foods for each mouthful	Do not work through each type of food on the plate separately
Establish a rhythm by observing how much time is needed for chewing and swallowing, checking with the person	Do not rush the person; make sure one mouthful is finished before offering another
Pause to offer drinks in between mouthfuls and to wipe mouth with a napkin	Do not scrape the spoon up a person's face to catch spills
After eating, help to wash and dry mouth and hands	Do not leave a person unattended at the table

Investigate

With another person, preferably a colleague, take it in turns to feed each other. Give each other feedback about the experience, noting what worked best and felt most comfortable.

Reflect

Try to imagine how it feels to be assisted with eating and what would improve the experience.

Discuss

Talk with colleagues about the different systems to help people with dementia keep their clothes, faces and hands clean at meal times. What are the advantages and disadvantages of each?

Case study

Winston, who is 85 and has dementia, lives alone but uses a care service that provides a carer at mealtimes to help him. He always coughs and splutters when he eats his food, sometimes making a mess down his front. One carer scolds him saying, 'I have to get you a new top every lunch time – you should be more careful'. On another occasion a different carer says, 'I'll feed you, then you won't choke and you won't spill anything'.

1. What is your response to the first carer's words?

2. What is your response to the second carer's words?

3. What would you say and do if you were a carer for Winston?

Knowledge Assessment Task

This assessment task covers DEM 302 2.1, 2.2, 2.3.

Mealtime cultures and environments can encourage or discourage eating, and it is the care worker's role to overcome barriers by working in a person-centred way. To complete this task, read through the scenarios and suggest strategies that reflect a person-centred approach to manage the situation.

1. *Bert often spills his meal down his front and his face becomes smeared with food. He screws his paper napkin into a ball and spits out the bits of food that are too difficult to chew. Bert's friend Tom sits with him and doesn't seem to mind, but his wife, who visits at lunchtime, makes derogatory comments about it being a monkey's tea-party and warns Tom to remember his manners.*

2. *Dilys has a 15-minute visit to prompt Mrs Vickery to eat the lunch provided by a meal service. She sets the table and calls her, but Mrs Vickery takes time to get to the table, visiting the toilet first and always wanting to chat, or show Dilys something. The 15 minutes is up before Mrs Vickery has started to eat sometimes, and the evening carers have reported finding unfinished meals.*

3. *Suki eats everything, whether it is food or not. She has eaten the flowers from a vase on the table and her paper napkin, and will empty the salt cellar into her mouth. She gets up and down from the table frequently and takes food from the plates of others. When she walks the corridors, care staff need to make sure nothing that could harm her is left out, because last week she was found trying to eat alcohol hand gel.*

Keep the written work that you produce as evidence for your assessment.

Supporting individuals with dementia to enjoy good nutrition

How can a person's life story guide the diet you provide?

Although the individuals you care for have probably had dementia all the time you have known them, they will have had a much longer, fuller and richer life before this. By finding out about this you will be able to:

- identify foods that hold meaning
- apply knowledge about the life story in order to meet preferences.

Identifying foods

Talk to a person during meal times – your conversation may provide information about their likes and dislikes. You can use pictures of food in magazines to prompt responses and look through illustrated recipe books together. Sometimes discussion about sources of food – for example the butcher's shop, the greengrocer and the baker, many of whom would have provided a door-to-door service – can stimulate memories.

Ask families and friends, who may have stories that spark memories about favourite meals. Some foods might not be familiar to you, but may still be available.

Applying life story

Use the information you uncover to inform the care you provide and share this with others on the team, making sure it is recorded. Include the person who decides menus and cooks the meals in your discussions, so that he or she understands the need for adjustments.

Pay attention to detail. For example, it isn't enough to know a person takes milk and sugar in coffee – how many spoonfuls? A splash of cold milk, or made with warm milk?

Look at figure 5.14 overleaf for more ideas.

Your assessment criteria:

DEM 302

3.1 Demonstrate how the knowledge of life history of an individual with dementia has been used to provide a diet that meets his or her preferences.

? Reflect

Think about your childhood and identify foods you feel nostalgic about – foods that comforted you or were part of celebrations. Those you provide care for will have their memories too, which can provide clues to meeting their dietary preferences.

Discuss

Talk with colleagues about practical methods for making sure information from life stories is used to inform care, making it individual to each person. Think about who needs to know the information, and where it should be recorded and displayed.

Investigate

Try an experiment with a person you provide care for: put bread in the toaster and while it is toasting, ask what the smell makes him or her think about and what memories it sparks. Try this with other aromas, such as vinegar, vanilla essence and lemon or orange zest.

How do you support the needs and abilities of individuals when they eat and drink?

It is important to organise meal times in ways that meet the specific needs and support the abilities of each individual you provide care for. Think particularly about:

- meal planning

- addressing needs and supporting abilities.

Meal planning

A regular timetable of meals, snacks and drinks will not necessarily suit each person with dementia, and it is important to tailor occasions for eating and drinking to the individual, rather than making them fit into a programme that suits you.

This flexible approach means you need to be sensitive to the best times, ways and environments to offer food and drink. Look at the diagram below (figure 5.14), which sets out the questions you need to be asking about each person for whom you provide care.

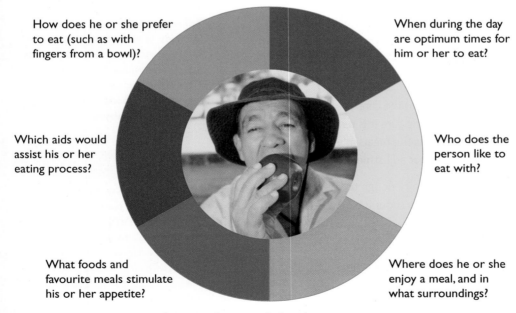

How does he or she prefer to eat (such as with fingers from a bowl)?

When during the day are optimum times for him or her to eat?

Which aids would assist his or her eating process?

Who does the person like to eat with?

What foods and favourite meals stimulate his or her appetite?

Where does he or she enjoy a meal, and in what surroundings?

Figure 5.14 Person-centred approach to meal planning

Case study

Frankie Ford worked in a fairground from the age of 14 until his twenties. The care workers discover this when someone mentions candy floss over the lunch table.

Frankie, who doesn't often say much, suddenly shouts out 'candy floss, toffee apples, fish 'n' chips and vinegar, whelks in a jar – that tickles my fancy!', and roars with laughter.

1. How can care workers use this information from Frankie's past?

2. How would you make sure this information was passed on?

3. How would you respond to a person who judges these foods to be 'nutritionally bad'?

Investigate

Find out whether there is a nutrition and nutritional screening policy where you work. If there is, read it and make sure you understand it. If there isn't, ask your manager about this.

Addressing needs and supporting abilities

It is just as important to recognise a person's abilities as it is to identify disabilities, so that you can build on strengths and help a person to remain independent for as long as possible. Look at the guidelines for addressing needs and supporting abilities in figure 5.15 below.

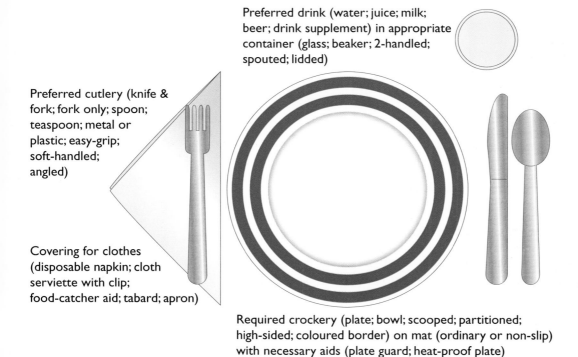

Figure 5.15 Guidelines for addressing needs and supporting abilities

How can you identify the positive effect of a person-centred approach on nutrition?

It is important to assess the impact of the care you give, to check it is meeting the needs and improving the wellbeing of each individual. To establish whether a person-centred approach is having a positive effect on nutrition you should consider:

- indicators of wellbeing
- weight measurements, BMI and MUST.

Indicators of wellbeing

It is important to observe, record and track a range of indicators for healthy nutrition. There is a danger too many charts can shift your attention from the person to the process of form-filling, so use the information you record to guide the care you give.

 Discuss

Discuss how to design a survey for service users and their family members to find out their opinions on menus, mealtime environments and practice.

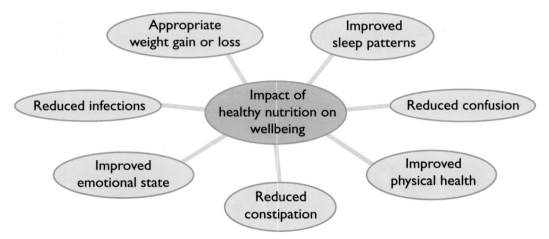

Figure 5.16 Indicators of improved health and wellbeing

Weight measurements, BMI and MUST

Weighing a person is a straightforward method of checking whether weight is stable. Doing this regularly allows comparisons to be made over time. The Body Mass Index (BMI) system looks at height and weight measurements together, compared across populations, and provides a scale indicating if a person is underweight (BMI under 18.5) or overweight (BMI over 30).

It may not be possible to weigh individuals in their own home, and some are unable to stand and balance sufficiently to use scales. In these cases you can use circumference measurements around the upper arm. This process is explained within a tool referred to as MUST, the Malnutrition Universal Screening Tool system. Information about this commonly used assessment tool will probably be available where you work, or can be accessed from the internet.

Investigate

Using work or internet sources, find out as much as you can about the MUST screening tool. Try it out on yourself to practise how to carry out the calculations accurately.

Case study

During a recent inspection of Balinrees care home, concern was expressed about the physical wellbeing of three residents who had each lost a significant amount of weight since admission. In response, the manager points out that measurements of weight were taken each month, the completed records proving there was no negligence.

1. In what ways do you think there might have been negligence?

2. Who would you inform if a person's weight measurements were changing?

3. What actions can be taken to stop unwanted weight loss, and how would you monitor progress?

? Reflect

How do you usually assess your own nutritional health? Think about the fit of your clothes; the appearance of skin, hair and nails; your energy levels; the way you feel about food and eating.

Discuss

Talk with colleagues about the different kinds of records that help you to keep track of a person's nutritional health and wellbeing.

Practical Assessment Task

This assessment task covers DEM 302 3.1, 3.4.

To be an effective care worker you must find out about each person as a unique individual and apply the information to provide a diet that suits preferences, meets nutritional requirements and improves wellbeing. To carry out this task you need to do the following.

1. *Select a person you work with who has dementia.*

2. *Create, or build on, a life story to highlight those elements that relate to dietary needs and preferences.*

3. *Write a care plan or draw a diagram that shows how you apply this information in practice to provide a diet that meets the nutritional requirements and personal preferences of the individual.*

4. *With reference to figure 5.16 opposite, provide evidence to show that wellbeing is improved by your interventions.*

Your evidence for this task must be based on your practice in a real work environment and must be presented in a format acceptable to your assessor.

Practical Assessment Task

This assessment task covers DEM 302 3.2, 3.3.

The mealtime environment and support for the abilities of each individual to eat and drink are as important as providing a healthy diet. Using the same person as for the previous task and with reference to figure 5.15 on page 195, carry out the following task.

1. *Draw your own meal setting plan to show how you intend to:*
   - *manage meal-, snack- and drink-time environments during a day for this person*
   - *support the person's eating and drinking abilities.*

2. *Identify the person's strengths and how you will build on these.*

3. *Identify aids and interventions required.*

Your evidence for this task must be based on your practice in a real work environment and must be presented in a format acceptable to your assessor.

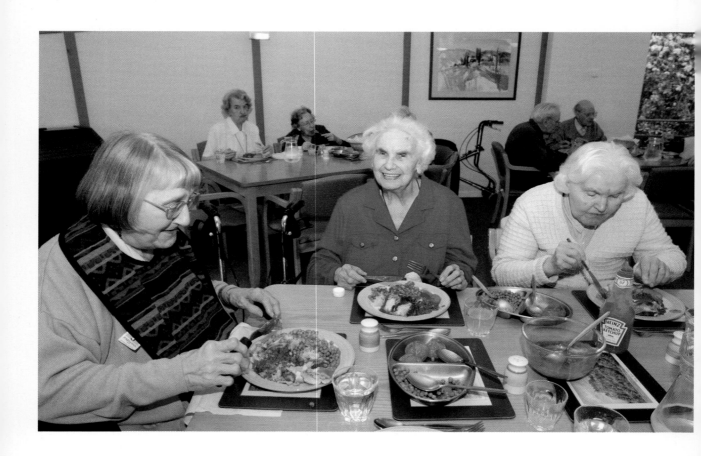

Assessment checklist

The assessment of this unit is partly knowledge-based (assessing things you need to know about) and partly competence-based (assessing things you need to do in the real work environment). To complete this unit successfully, you will need to produce evidence of both your knowledge and your competence.

The knowledge-based assessment criteria for DEM 302 are listed in the 'What you need to know' table below. The practical or competence-based criteria for DEM 302 are listed in the 'What you need to do' table below. Your tutor or assessor will help you to prepare for your assessment, and the tasks suggested in the chapter will help you to create the evidence you need.

Assessment criteria	What you need to know	Assessment task
DEM 302		
1.1	Describe how cognitive, functional and emotional changes associated with dementia can affect eating, drinking and nutrition	Page 178
1.2	Explain how poor nutrition can contribute to an individual's experience of dementia	Page 178
1.3	Outline how other health and emotional conditions may affect the nutritional needs of an individual with dementia	Page 178
1.4	Explain the importance of recognising and meeting an individual's personal and cultural preferences for food and drink	Page 185
1.5	Explain why it is important to include a variety of food and drink in the diet of an individual with dementia	Page 185
2.1	Describe how mealtime cultures and environments can be a barrier to meeting the nutritional needs of an individual with dementia	Page 192
2.2	Describe how mealtime environments and food presentation can be designed to help an individual to eat and drink	Page 192
2.3	Describe how a person-centred approach can support an individual, with dementia at different levels of ability, to eat and drink	Page 192

Assessment criteria	What you need to do	Assessment task
3.1	Demonstrate how the knowledge of life history of an individual with dementia has been used to provide a diet that meets his/her preferences	Page 197
3.2	Demonstrate how meal times for an individual with dementia are planned to support his/her ability to eat and drink	Page 198
3.3	Demonstrate how the specific eating and drinking abilities and needs of an individual with dementia have been addressed	Page 198
3.4	Demonstrate how a person-centred approach to meeting nutritional requirements has improved the wellbeing of an individual with dementia	Page 197

Resources

Services and organisations

The organisations listed below provide information, guidance and a range of care and support services that address the needs of individuals with dementia as well as the people who provide care and support for them. (All information correct at time of going to press.)

Organisation	Website	Description
Alzheimer's Association	www.alz.org/AboutAD/Stages.asp	The leading USA-based voluntary organisation for information on Alzheimer's care
Alzheimer's Disease International	www.alz.co.uk/carers/yourself.html	An umbrella organisation representing Alzheimer's organisations around the world. It seeks to raise awareness of Alzheimer's and other causes of dementia
Alzheimer's Research UK	www.alzheimers-research.org.uk	The leading UK charity of research into the cure, prevention and treatment of Alzheimer's and other forms of dementia
Alzheimer Scotland	www.alzscot.org/	The leading voluntary organisation in Scotland that supports and works on behalf of people with dementia, their carers and families
Alzheimer Scotland: Dementia Rights	www.dementiarights.org	Alzheimer Scotland's campaign for the rights of people with dementia and their carers. The site includes lots of useful information about equality, rights and discrimination that applies to the UK as well as Scotland
Alzheimer's Society	www.alzheimers.org.uk/site/index.php	A leading UK research and care charity for people with dementia, their families and carers
AT Dementia	www.atdementia.org.uk	Information on assistive technology for people with dementia
Bradford Dementia Group	www.brad.ac.uk/acad/health/dementia	Information about research, education and training that aims to improve quality of life and care for people with dementia and their families
Dementia Advocacy Support Network (DASN) International	www.dasninternational.org	A global support network that promotes respect, dignity and support for people with dementia
Dementia Awareness	www.dementiaawareness.co.uk	A group that campaigns to raise awareness of dementia. The site provides useful information and valuable insights into the experiences of individuals with dementia and their carers
Dementia Cafe	www.dementiacentre.com	An online space for people with dementia, their families and carers as well as professionals. The site allows you to give and receive information and support about dementia-related issues
Dementia UK	www.dementiauk.com	This website promotes and seeks to develop the work of Admiral Nurses in the UK. These are specialist nurses who focus on meeting the needs of the carers and families of individuals with dementia
Mental Health Foundation	www.mentalhealth.org.uk/information/mental-health-a-z/dementia/	This site provides information and resources about dementia and care-related issues

Organisation	Website	Description
National Institute of Clinical Excellence (NICE)	www.nice.org.uk	This organisation provides information about standards and best practice in dementia care. To find out more, type 'Dementia' into the website's search feature
NHS Choices	www.nhs.uk	Information and links to other sites on a wide range of health and care issues that are relevant to people with dementia and their families
Royal College of Nursing	www.rcn.org.uk	This organisation represents nurses and nursing and provides a range of information and publications on or relevant to dementia care issues
Social Care Institute for Excellence (SCIE)	www.scie.org.uk/ publications/dementia	An independent charity that works with a range of vulnerable individuals, carers and service providers to raise awareness of social care issues. SCIE campaign on dementia care issues and produce a range of useful publications
Talking Point	http://forum.alzheimers.org. uk/forum.php	The Alzheimer's Society online forum for individuals with dementia, their carers and family members

Further reading

Further reading on a wide variety of issues covered in this handbook can be found in the publications listed below.

Adams T. and Clarke C. L. (Eds) *Dementia Care: Developing Partnerships in Practice*. Bailliere Tindall 1999

Bartle, C. *Knowledge Set for Dementia*. Heinemann 2007

Bayley, J. *Iris: A Memoir of Iris Murdoch*. Abacus 1999

Bhugra, D. and Bahl, V. *Ethnicity: An Agenda for Mental Health*. Gaskell 1999

Bryden, C. *Dancing with Dementia*. Jessica Kingsley 2005

Davis, R. *My Journey into Alzheimer's Disease*. Tyndale House 1989

Downs, M. *Excellence in Dementia Care*. Open University Press 2008

Feil, N. *The Validation Breakthrough*. Barnes and Noble 2002

Friel-McGowin, D. *Living in the Labyrinth: A Personal Journey Through the Maze of Alzheimer's Disease*. Delacorte Press 1993

Goldsmith, M. *Hearing the Voice of People with Dementia: Opportunities and Obstacles*. Jessica Kingsley 1996

Kerr, D. *Understanding Learning Disabilities and Dementia – Developing Effective Interventions*. Jessica Kingsley 2005

Killick, J. and Allan, K. *Communication and the Care of Older People with Dementia*. Open University Press 2002

Kitwood, T. *Dementia Reconsidered*. Open University Press 1997

Morris, G. and Morris, J. *The Dementia Care Workbook*. Open University Press/McGraw Hill 2010

Pritchard, J. *Good Practice in the Law and Safeguarding Adults – Criminal Justice and Adult Protection*. Jessica Kingsley 2008

Schweitzer, P. and Bruce, E. *Remembering Yesterday, Caring Today – Reminiscence in Dementia Care: A Guide to Good Practice*. Jessica Kingsley 2008

Social Care Institute for Excellence, *Assessing the Mental Health Needs of Older People*. www.scie.org.uk/publications 2006

Sutcliffe, D. *Introducing Dementia – The Essential Facts and Issues of Care*. Age Concern England 2001

Index

Acknowledgements

Every effort has been made to trace copyright holders and to obtain their permission for the use of copyright material. The publishers will gladly receive any information enabling them to rectify any error or omission at the first opportunity.

The publishers would like to thank the following for permission to reproduce photographs:

(t = top, b = bottom, c = centre, l = left, r = right)

Cover & p i: Stuart Key/Dreamstime.com; pp4–5: Lisa F. Young/Shutterstock; p6: Science Photo Library; p9: Brian Eichhorn/Shutterstock; p11:Konstantin Sutyagin/Shutterstock; p12l: Petr Nad/Shutterstock; p12r: Juice Images/Alamy; p14: Lisa S./Shutterstock; p16: Monkey Business Images/Shutterstock; p19: Jim Lopes/Shutterstock; p21: Medical-on-Line/Alamy; p24: Mira Alamy; p26: Vinicius Tupinamba/Shutterstock; p27: Goodluz/Shutterstock; p28: Adrian Sherratt/Alamy; p30: Corbis Premium RF/Alamy; p31: Peter Titmuss/Alamy; p32: Monkey Business Images; pp34–37:Gilles Lougassi/Shutterstock; p38: Michal Bednarek/Shutterstock; p41: Sturti/iStock; p43: MBI Alamy; p45: Paul Doyle/Alamy; p46: Andres Balcazar/ iStock; p49: MBI/Alamy; p53: Paula Solloway/Alamy; p55: Andresr/Shutterstock; p57: David Levenson/Alamy; p58: Dean Mitchell/iStock; p60: Lise Dumont/Alamy; p62: Monkey Business Images/Shutterstock; p64: Imagebroker/Alamy; p67: Ed Bock/Shutterstock; p69: Ed Phillips/Shutterstock; pp74–77: Catherine Yeulet/ iStock; p78: Stockbroker/Alamy; p84: Paul Doyle/Alamy; p86: Caro/Alamy; p90: David Taylor/Alamy; p92: Tetra Images/Alamy; p93: Radius Images/Alamy; p98: Tetra Images/Alamy; p99: 67photo/Alamy; p103: Art Kowalsky/Alamy; p107: Corbis Bridge/Alamy; p108: Blend Images/Alamy; p109: Kumar Sriskandan/ Alamy; p110: Pamela Moore/iStock; p114: Nancy Louie/iStock; p115: Bubbles Photolibrary/Alamy; p117: Paula Solloway/Alamy; p118: Catchlight Visual Services/ Alamy; p119: Juice Images/Alamy; pp126–129: Mangostock/Shutterstock; p132: Dan White/Alamy; p134: Dinga/Shutterstock; p137: James Steidl/Shutterstock; p138: Ramona Heim/Shutterstock; p140: Monkey Business Images/Shutterstock; p141: Maskot/Alamy; p144: Olivier Le Queinec/Shutterstock; p145: Arkady/ Shutterstock; p146: Kuzma/Shutterstock; p148: Daniel M. Nagy/Shutterstock; p151t: Absolut/Shutterstock; p151b: Creatista/Shutterstock; p153: Paul Doyle/ Alamy; p154: Golden Pixels LLC/Shutterstock; p156: Chris Schmidt/iStock; p157: Penny Tweedie/Alamy; p159: Custom Medical Stock Photo/Alamy; p160: Kacso Sandor/Shutterstock; p161: Yuri Arcurs/Shutterstock; p163: TravelStockCollection - Homer Sykes/Alamy; p165: Jason Stitt/Shutterstock; pp170–171: Monkey Business Images/Shutterstock; p172: David Hoffman/Alamy; p173: Moodboard/Alamy; p176: Simone van den Berg/Shutterstock; p178: Jodi Jacobson/iStock; p181: Blaj Gabriel/Shutterstock; p182: Corbis Flirt/Alamy; p184: Helen Sessions/Alamy; p187: Alexander Raths/iStock; p190: Stockbroker/Alamy; p194: GlowImages/Alamy; p198: Jack Sullivan/Alamy.

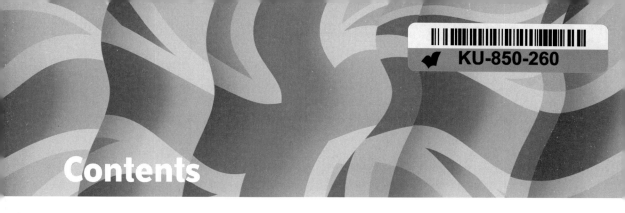

Contents

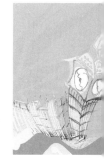

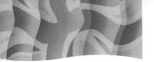

Annual Survey 2010

UK Government & Politics

Paul Fairclough

Eric Magee

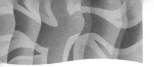

Philip Allan Updates, an imprint of Hodder Education, part of Hachette UK, Market Place, Deddington, Oxfordshire OX15 0SE

Orders
Bookpoint Ltd, 130 Milton Park, Abingdon, Oxfordshire OX14 4SB
tel: 01235 827720
fax: 01235 400454
e-mail: uk.orders@bookpoint.co.uk

Lines are open 9.00 a.m.–5.00 p.m., Monday to Saturday, with a 24-hour message answering service. You can also order through the Philip Allan Updates website: www.philipallan.co.uk

© Philip Allan Updates 2010

ISBN 978-1-4441-1043-2

First published 2010
Impression number   5   4   3   2   1
Year   2014   2013   2012   2011   2010

Printed by MPG Books, Bodmin

Hachette UK's policy is to use papers that are natural, renewable and recyclable products and made from wood grown in sustainable forests. The logging and manufacturing processes are expected to conform to the environmental regulations of the country of origin.

Chapter 1

Election roundup: Labour in freefall?

Context

Although there were fewer by-elections in 2009 than in 2008, the year still provided a number of opportunities for the main UK parties to test their electoral strength ahead of a likely general election in May 2010. The New Year provided an opportunity for New Labour to move on from what had been something of an *annus horribilis* at the polls in 2008 — with the party suffering significant losses in the local elections held on 1 May as well as failing to secure victory in four of the five by-elections held in the year: losing the seats of Crewe and Nantwich and Glasgow East; and slipping to fifth place in Henley, behind both the Green Party and British National Party candidates.

This chapter considers the extent to which Labour's victory at the Glenrothes by-election in November 2008 was anything more than a fleeting pause in the party's freefall towards defeat at the 2010 general election. In so doing it will address questions such as:

- How well did Labour perform in the 2009 local elections?
- What factors prompted the two by-elections held in 2009, what issues were they fought on and how well did Labour perform?
- What, if anything, can we learn from the 2009 elections to the European Parliament?
- Is New Labour now incapable of winning the next general election?

How well did Labour perform in the 2009 local elections?

Whereas the local government elections held in May 2008 had mainly involved unitary authorities and second-tier authorities (i.e. borough and district councils) in England and Wales, 2009 saw seats on all 27 English county councils contested. That distinction aside, the verdict we delivered in our 2009 survey still largely rings true (see Box 1.1).

Box 1.1 A case of déjà vu?

Although attempts to extrapolate results in local elections onto a bigger electoral canvas are fraught with problems, such extensive losses would certainly have given Labour pause for thought: not least because those losing their seats in such contests are the very grassroots activists upon whose shoulders falls the burden of organising the general election campaign at constituency level. Such reversals at the polls are not, therefore, simply about losing control of local councils: they can also represent a degrading of the local party infrastructure.

Source: P. Fairclough and E. Magee, *UK Government and Politics Annual Survey 2009*, Phillip Allan Updates.

While it is not uncommon for a party in government to experience heavy losses at local elections — not least as a result of the increased prevalence of protest voting common at such second-order elections — the scale of Labour's losses in recent years has effectively seen the party wiped out as a force in local government in many parts of the UK. This erosion of party representation at the grassroots level has implications that go beyond the 'degrading of the local party infrastructure' we identified in 2009, because it also has implications for political recruitment at the national level. The pool from which the Labour Party has traditionally selected its prospective parliamentary candidates has, in effect, been halved in size in little more than a decade. Yet the alternative — namely to select candidates who have no experience of grassroots party activity — threatens the very principles upon which the Labour Party was founded, as well as contributing to the growing sense that the Commons has become a playground for a generation of professional politicians, fast-tracked through from university to high office.

The scale of the party's losses in 2009 (see Table 1.1) brings to mind the experience of John Major's Conservatives as they limped towards a record defeat at the 1997 general election. Back in 1996 the Conservatives secured just 29% of the vote at the local elections (Labour 43%, Liberal Democrats 24%) before going on to secure a disappointing 30.7% at the general election the following year (Labour 43.2%, Liberal Democrats 16.8%). If anything, the 2009 local elections saw Labour fare worse than the Conservatives had done 13 years earlier: the party was pushed into third place with just 23% of the popular vote (Conservatives 38%, Liberal Democrats 28%).

Table 1.1 Local election performance compared: 2008 and 2009

Party	1 May 2008: England and Wales Councils Net +/−	Total	Councillors Net +/−	Total	4 June 2009: England Councils Net +/−	Total	Councillors Net +/−	Total
Conservative	12	65	257	3,155	7	30	244	1,531
Labour	−9	18	−334	2,365	−4	0	−291	178
Liberal Democrat	1	12	33	1,804	−1	1	−2	484
Others	−1	0	41	1,092	0	0	41	169
No overall control	−3	64	–	–	−2	3	–	–
	159 councils declared				27 councils declared			

Source: figures taken from www.bbc.co.uk, May 2008 and May 2009.

Mayoral contests
The three contests for directly elected mayors held in 2009 — in Doncaster, Hartlepool and North Tyneside — offered little comfort for New Labour. In North Tyneside, the incumbent Labour mayor, John Harrison, was defeated by the Conservative candidate, Linda Arkley. In Doncaster and Hartlepool the trend for such elections to throw up quirky winners continued, with the

English Democrat candidate, Peter Davies, returned in Doncaster and the one-time Hartlepool Football Club mascot Stuart Drummond (aka H'Angus the Monkey) returned for a third consecutive term as mayor of Hartlepool.

What factors prompted the two by-elections held in 2009, what issues were they fought on and how well did Labour perform?

There have now been 14 by-elections since the 2005 general election (see Table 1.2), with many of those held in the last 2 years arising not as a result of the death of the incumbent MP — as is commonly the case — but in the wake of a resignation. The two by-elections that took place in 2009, in Norwich North and Glasgow North East, both fell into this category.

Table 1.2 By-elections, 2005–09

Constituency	Date	Cause
Cheadle	14 July 2005	Death
Livingston	29 September 2005	Death
Dunfermline and West Fife	9 February 2006	Death
Blaenau Gwent	29 June 2006	Death
Bromley and Chislehurst	29 June 2006	Death
Ealing Southall	19 July 2007	Death
Sedgefield	19 July 2007	Resignation
Crewe and Nantwich	22 May 2008	Death
Henley	26 June 2008	Resignation
Haltemprice and Howden	10 July 2008	Resignation
Glasgow East	24 July 2008	Resignation
Glenrothes	6 November 2008	Death
Norwich North	23 July 2009	Resignation
Glasgow North East	12 November 2009	Resignation

Norwich North (27 July)

Although Labour's landslide defeat at the Norwich North by-election led to talk of electoral wipeout for the party at the 2010 general election, closer analysis of the result reveals that the loss of the seat might not have any great electoral significance beyond that constituency (Table 1.3, p. 4).

What prompted the by-election?

The by-election was prompted by the decision of the sitting Labour MP, Ian Gibson, to resign after being told that he would not be permitted to stand as a candidate for the party at the next election following the furore over MPs expenses. Specifically, he was being de-selected because of the way in which he had allegedly profited from the sale of a property he had in part paid for using his MP's second homes allowance.

Chapter 1

Table 1.3 Norwich North by-election: Conservative gain

Party	General election: 5 May 2005		By-election: 27 July 2009	
	Votes	%	Votes	%
Labour	21,097	44.0	6,243	18.2
Conservative	15,638	33.2	13,591	39.5
Liberal Democrat	7,616	16.2	4,803	14.0
Green	1,252	2.7	3,350	9.7
UKIP	1,122	2.4	4,068	11.8
Others (7 candidates)	308	0.7	2,322	6.8
Turnout	61.1%		45.9%	
Swing	16.5% (Labour to Conservative)			

What issues was it fought on?

While the election was widely seen as a verdict on Labour's performance in office, the campaign was fought against the backdrop of the expenses row, with Labour supporters in the constituency apparently harbouring considerable sympathy for the 'ousted' MP. The Conservatives chose the 27 year-old former business advisor Chloe Smith as their candidate. Although the selection of such a young, female candidate clearly fitted David Cameron's stated desire to broaden the range of candidates adopted by the party — as seen in his experiments with A-lists and primary elections (see UK Update, *Politics Review*, Vol. 19, No. 2) — this was not the key factor in the contest, as evidenced by the result.

How well did Labour perform?

Gordon Brown's verdict on the result in Norwich North was that it was a bad day for all three of the main parties: they had all lost votes compared to their performance at the 2005 general election. Brown's take on the result ignored the fact that the Conservatives had in fact increased their share of the vote in the face of a massively reduced turnout. However, the prime minister's observations hinted at larger truths: first, that smaller parties had made major gains; and second, that the Conservatives' victory came not as a result of a massive increase in their own support, but as a consequence of the collapse of the Labour vote. This collapse in Labour's support within the constituency was generally agreed to have been a direct result of the party's treatment of Gibson, with many Labour voters opting to stay at home in protest at the *de facto* de-selection of their constituency MP.

Glasgow North East (12 November)

What prompted the by-election?

The by-election in Glasgow North East resulted from similar circumstances to those that had prompted the contest in Norwich North 4 months earlier: the incumbent MP and former speaker of the House of Commons, Michael

Martin, resigned in the wake of criticism of his handling of the row over MPs' expenses. In other respects, however, the contest was unusual.

What issues was it fought on?

By convention, the mainstream opposition parties do not field candidates against a sitting speaker. As a result, the Conservatives and Liberal Democrats had never contested Glasgow North East and had not fought in the constituency it replaced — Glasgow Springburn — since 1997. They were therefore starting at a distinct disadvantage in 2009.

The result was a contest that centred on the relative merits of the Labour candidate (and by implication the Labour government at Westminster) and the SNP candidate and the party's minority administration at Holyrood. Although local issues such as rising unemployment were also well to the fore, the campaign was not sufficiently dynamic to move many of those registered to vote to actually cast a ballot, with turnout falling to just 33.2% (see Table 1.4).

Table 1.4 Glasgow North East by-election: Labour hold

Party	General election: 5 May 2008		By-election: 12 November 2009	
	Votes	%	Votes	%
Speaker/Labour	**15,153**	**53.3**	**12,231**	**59.4**
SNP	5,019	17.7	4,120	20.0
Others (11 candidates)	8,246	29	4,244	20.6
Turnout	45.8%		33.2%	

How well did Labour perform?

Although Labour retained the seat in a contest that rendered any calculation of swing pointless, the question of what precisely can be learnt from such a victory is far harder to answer. Just as Labour's victory at Glenrothes 12 months earlier proved to be nothing more than a blip in the party's downward electoral spiral, it is difficult to measure Labour's performance against its two main rivals at the next general election in a contest in which neither stood any realistic chance of being well placed.

What, if anything, can we learn from the 2009 elections to the European Parliament?

The 2009 elections to the European Parliament saw Labour pushed into third place in the polls (see Tables 1.5 and 1.6). This was, as we have seen, the same fate it suffered in the local elections held on the same day — though here it trailed UKIP as opposed to the Liberal Democrats. UKIP's performance at the polls came as a surprise to those who had predicted that the party would struggle to hold onto the 12 seats it had won with the broadcaster Robert Kilroy Silk fronting its campaign back in 2004. In the event, the party not only

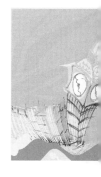

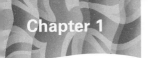

increased its share of the popular vote, but also increased the number of seats it won from 12 to 13: this in an election at which the UK was only returning 72 MEPs to the European Parliament (69 from Great Britain, 3 from Northern Ireland) as opposed to the 78 (75 + 3) elected 4 years earlier.

Table 1.5 2009 elections to the European Parliament in Great Britain

Party	Votes (%)	Change (+/–)	MEPs (69)	Change (+/–)
Conservative	4,198,394 (27.7%)	+1.0%	25	+1
UKIP	2,498,226 (16.5%)	+0.3%	13	+1
Labour	2,381,760 (15.7%)	–6.9%	13	-5
Liberal Democrat	2,080,613 (13.7%)	–1.2%	11	+1
Green	1,223,303 (8.6%)	+2.4%	2	0
BNP	943,598 (6.2%)	+1.3%	2	+2
SNP	321,007 (2.1%)	+0.7%	2	0
Plaid Cymru	126,702 (0.8%)	–0.1%	1	0
Others	1,298,722 (8.6%)	–	–	–
Turnout	34.0%			

Table 1.6 2009 elections to the European Parliament in Northern Ireland

Candidate	Party	First preferences Votes	%	MEPs (3)	Change (+/–)
Bairbre de Brún	Sinn Féin	126,184	25.8	1	0
Diane Dodds	Democratic Unionist	88,346	18.1	1	0
Jim Nicholson	Ulster Conservatives and Unionists	82,892	17.0	1	0
Alban Maginness	Social Democratic and Labour	78,489	16.1	0	0
	Others	108,660	22.2	0	0
	Turnout	42.8%			

Elections to the European Parliament have in the past proven to be notoriously bad predictors of general election performance. This is a consequence not only of the proportional systems adopted in such contests since 1999, but also the far higher levels of protest voting witnessed in them. In 2009 such protest voting was further fuelled by ongoing concerns over the Lisbon Treaty and the UK referendum that wasn't (see Chapter 5).

What is clear, however, is that the 2009 European elections provided a real boost for the larger minor parties ahead of the next general election. The Greens won two seats — just as they had in both 2004 and 1999 (the year when a proportional system was first employed) and UKIP consolidated its position after major gains in 2004. Perhaps most notable, however, was the success enjoyed by the BNP, with the party winning two seats: Andrew Brons being elected in the Yorkshire and the Humber region with 9.8% of the vote; and the party's leader, Nick Griffin, returned with 8.0% of the vote in the North West England region.

The knock-on effects of this, the BNP's first major electoral success aside from it winning a seat on the 25-member Greater London Assembly back in 2008, are too far-reaching to consider in detail here. Suffice to say, it will result in a major boost to the party's finances and also make it more likely that its representatives will enjoy more air-time than has been the case previously, as seen with Nick Griffin's controversial appearance on the BBC's *Question Time* programme on 22 October 2009.

Conclusions: is New Labour now incapable of winning the next general election?

Although the Labour Party's performance at elections in 2009 did little to suggest that it would be capable of mounting a serious challenge at the next general election, the end of the year did sound one or two notes of caution for those hoping for an end to the Conservative Party's 13 years in opposition.

While Labour's victory at the Glasgow North East by-election may prove to be nothing more than a temporary diversion on its path out of office — like its success at Glenrothes a year earlier — the closing weeks of 2009 did see the party making progress in the opinion polls (see Box 1.2). Although these same polls showed Gordon Brown's personal approval rating running at an alarming –25 points, this was a full 17-point improvement on the figure recorded back in July 2009.

Box 1.2	Grounds for optimism?

Q1a How would you vote if there were a general election tomorrow?

If undecided or refused at Q1a:

Q1b Which party are you most inclined to support?

Party	Q1a/b November (October) 2009
Conservative	37% (43%)
Labour	31% (26%)
Liberal Democrats	17% (19%)
Scottish/Welsh Nationalist	3% (4%)
Green Party	3% (2%)
UK Independence Party	3% (2%)
British National Party	2% (1%)
Other	4% (2%)

Source: adapted from Ipsos MORI Political Monitor.

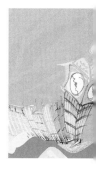

The parallels between New Labour's fortunes over the last 12 months and what happened to the Conservatives ahead of their defeat at the 1997 general election are all too obvious. For the Conservatives, however, the fear must be that far from seeing a repeat of the 12 months that preceded the 1997 general election, we are in fact witnessing something akin to what happened in the run-up to the general election in 1992, when a party apparently on course for victory after a lengthy period in opposition somehow managed to snatch defeat from the jaws of victory.

Summary

- In 2009 the Labour Party suffered extensive losses in both the local elections and the European Parliament elections held on 4 June.
- The party was pushed into third place in both contests — trailing behind the Liberal Democrats in the local elections and UKIP in elections to the European Parliament.
- The two by-elections held in 2009 brought better news for Labour. Its defeat in Norwich North resulted more from unhappiness among its own voters than from any growth in support for the Conservatives, and it 'retained' Glasgow North East comfortably with an increased majority (35.7% up to 39.4%).
- Labour's plight at the end of 2009 brought to mind the problems that faced John Major's Conservative Party as it headed towards defeat at the 1997 general election.
- The publication of more favourable poll findings in some newspapers towards the end of 2009 sounded a note of caution for the Conservatives, while offering a glimmer of hope for New Labour.

Chapter 2

David Cameron: ready for power?

Context

By the time that many of you come to read this survey, the 2010 general election will already have taken place and David Cameron will, in all probability, have been installed at No 10. However, while it is one thing to make a party in opposition for more than a decade electable once more, it is quite another to govern once that elusive election victory has been secured.

This chapter considers whether David Cameron has the qualities to be prime minister. In so doing it will address the following questions:
- Does Cameron have the necessary abilities and experience?
- Does Cameron have 'the vision thing'?
- Will Cameron be able to carry the general public with him?
- What potential pitfalls will face Cameron if he becomes prime minister?

Does Cameron have the necessary abilities and experience?

Although individual prime ministers necessarily take different routes to No 10, all at some point face questions regarding their qualifications to serve in that office. Our initial verdict on Gordon Brown, delivered in our 2008 survey (see Box 2.1), was that while the Member for Kirkcaldy and Cowdenbeath was certainly intellectually capable and had performed creditably in the post of chancellor of the exchequer, he perhaps lacked some of the skills demanded of a modern premier; most notably in his dealings with cabinet colleagues and the media.

Box 2.1	Our initial verdict on Brown

It is clearly far too early to judge just how effective a prime minister Gordon Brown may eventually become. What is clear, however, is that 10 years spent as chancellor — shielded from the full glare of media attention by a prime minister who revelled in it — has afforded the former chancellor little opportunity to develop the full range of skills he will need to succeed in the top job. Though the thoroughness and determination Brown demonstrated when chancellor have afforded him a certain amount of political capital, modern political leadership requires a clearer and more compelling vision than the prime minister has, as yet, been able to articulate.

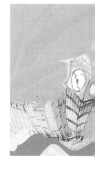

Source: P. Fairclough and E. Magee, *UK Government and Politics Annual Survey 2008*, Philip Allan Updates.

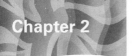

When assessing the extent to which David Cameron is ready to take on the mantle of chief executive it is perhaps more appropriate to compare his credentials with those of Tony Blair as opposed to Brown, for reasons that will become apparent.

Intellectual abilities

Cameron, like Blair, was educated at a leading independent school (see Table 2.1) before going on to study at Oxford. Though academic achievement is no prerequisite for high office (John Major being a case in point), the path trodden by Cameron is one shared with countless other leading politicians, past and present. Indeed, Eton has traditionally been seen as the 'chief nurse of England's statesmen', having educated 18 former prime ministers. Although Cameron was not fast-tracked through secondary education and on to university at the age of 16 — the case with Gordon Brown — the Conservative leader's effortless First at Oxford marks him out as a man of high intellectual ability.

Experience in office

Blair took on the mantle of leader of the opposition in 1994, just 11 years after being elected to represent the parliamentary constituency of Sedgefield for the first time. Though he had served in the shadow cabinet prior to his election as party leader, Blair had no experience in government office prior to becoming prime minister in 1997. Cameron had been an MP for just 4 years when he defeated David Davis in the run-off to become Conservative leader in 2005. Like Blair, he has never held ministerial office. Should the Conservatives be returned to government in 2010, Cameron will have made the journey from prospective parliamentary candidate to prime minister in just 9 years; 2 years short of the mark set by John Major. Although Cameron served as a special advisor in the last Conservative administration, he would surely be one of the least experienced incumbents at No 10 in the modern era should his party prevail at the polls. However, he will have served as leader of the opposition for 2 years longer than Tony Blair did prior to New Labour's victory at the 1997 general election.

The ability to engage with the public at large

Though Labour has attempted to brand Cameron and his inner circle as a clique of Eton-educated 'Tory toffs', the Conservative leader has in fact proven incredibly adept at reaching out to those beyond his immediate social class. Cameron is clearly at ease in the media spotlight — much as Blair was — and this is in marked contrast to both Brown (as we saw in our 2009 survey) and, to a lesser degree, David Davis; the man Cameron defeated to become Conservative leader back in 2005. This is surely not pure happenstance. The decision of rank-and-file Conservative Party members to lend their support to Cameron in the run-off ballot was seen by many as that party's 'Blair moment', a realisation that the party needed to look beyond more conventional choices and select a leader who was capable of reaching out to those who had stopped voting Conservative in the 1990s — something party members had singularly failed to grasp when choosing Iain Duncan Smith over Kenneth Clarke in 2001.

The ability to carry his party with him

It is a fact that political parties that have endured a lengthy period in opposition are more open to new ideas and approaches. Blair's rebranding of Labour from 1994, the reform of Clause 4 and the introduction of one-member-one-vote would have been far harder to execute had the party not suffered four successive general election defeats in 1979, 1983, 1987 and 1992. Cameron took up the reins of the Conservative Party when it was at a similar point in the political cycle; having fallen short in 1997 (under Major), 2001 (under Hague) and 2005 (under Howard). In a sense, therefore, the task of keeping the party in line is made easier by a collective sense that maintaining a united front in public — however unpalatable that might be — represents the only route back into government. Such a sense of unity and purpose is likely to continue into government, though papered-over divisions over Europe (particularly in light of the Irish and Polish ratification of the Lisbon Treaty) and other issues are likely to emerge at some point thereafter.

Table 2.1 Paths to No 10

Name	School	University	MP	Cabinet experience	PM
Margaret Thatcher	Kesteven and Grantham Girls' School (State grammar)	Oxford	Finchley (1959–92)	Education and science (1970–74)	1979–90
John Major	Rutlish Grammar School (State grammar)	–	Huntingdon (1983–2001) Huntingdonshire (1979–83)	Chief secretary to the Treasury (1987–88) Foreign secretary (1989) Chancellor of the exchequer (1989–90)	1990–97
Tony Blair	Fettes College (Independent boarding)	Oxford	Sedgefield (1983–2007)	–	1997–2007
Gordon Brown	Kirkcaldy High School (State grammar)	Edinburgh	Kirkcaldy and Cowdenbeath (2005–) Dunfermline East (1983–2005)	Chancellor of the exchequer (1997–2007)	2007–
David Cameron	Eton (Independent boarding)	Oxford	Witney (2001–)	–	–

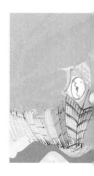

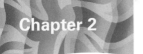
Does Cameron have 'the vision thing'?

Though electoral success can be based, to a degree at least, on negative sentiment — a reaction against a party too long in office — it is hard to establish anything of real worth unless one can articulate some kind of coherent vision as to where one wants to take the country.

In this respect it is probably fair to say that 'the jury is still out' on Cameron's time as Conservative leader.

In a piece entitled 'Conservatism under Cameron' in *Politics Review*, Vol. 17, No. 3 (2008), Richard Kelly offered three possible perspectives on Cameron's conservatism:
- *first*, that it represented a 'flagrant capitulation to New Labour'
- *second*, that it should be seen as a 'subtle continuation of Thatcherism'
- *third*, that it amounted to little more than 'shameless opportunism'

There are elements of truth in all three judgements on the approach Cameron has taken since becoming party leader, but it is the last that presents the biggest obstacle as he looks to move the Conservatives from the mentality of a party in opposition to that of a party in power.

The triumph of spin over substance?

In many policy areas well-received rhetoric has simply not been followed up with substantive policy detail; a failing forgivable in a party in opposition but less so in one so close to taking up the reins of power. Talk of replacing the Human Rights Act (1998) with a new British Bill of Rights has yet to move beyond the drawing board — a criticism that could be levelled at Cameron's democratic reform agenda as a whole (see Box 2.2), despite the party's experiment with a fully open primary in Totnes ('UK Update', *Politics Review*, Vol. 19, No. 2).

Box 2.2   Substance or spin?

David Cameron has sought to engage with the democratic reform agenda in a way that no Conservative leader has done before. Early in his leadership, he spoke at the Power Inquiry conference, hailing the Power Report as 'one of the most important initiatives we've seen for many years'. Last year his chapter in *Unlocking Democracy: 20 Years of Charter 88* stated that 'the Conservative Party's ambition is to restore engagement and promote accountability so that we can build trust in the political system'.

What will Cameron do over the next few months to ensure that his claim to embody change amounts to more than mere rhetoric? Having welcomed the Power Inquiry, for example, will he now engage constructively with Power2010? If he doesn't, he may well find that like Tony Blair, his words in opposition will come back to haunt him.

Source: P. Facey, 'David Cameron — change we can trust?', *Guardian*, 5 October 2009.

The party's position on taxation appears similarly opaque. Back in 2007 the emphasis was on bringing back the married person's allowance (even extending it to same-sex couples in civil partnerships) and raising the threshold for inheritance tax — an announcement that wrong-footed Labour and was said to have contributed to Brown's decision not to call a snap election that autumn. By the time of the 2009 party conference, however, the focus had switched to state pensions and public sector pay cuts. While the unravelling global credit crisis has clearly played a part in reordering the party's priorities, some have criticised a tendency to issue policy statements for short-term effect without really taking the time to consider the mid- to long-term consequences of what is being proposed (see Box 2.3).

Box 2.3 Policy on the hoof?

George Osborne will today announce at Conference that the Conservatives would increase the pension age from 65 to 66 by 2016 as opposed to 2026, as envisaged by the government.

However, analysts have immediately spotted a problem. The Labour government has already been raising the retirement age for women, bringing it in line with that for men, but this process will not be completed until 2020. Were the Conservatives to stick with their 2016 they would in effect be raising the pension age for women from 63 to 66 in a single year.

Source: P. Wintour and A. Sparrow, 'David Cameron forced to clarify retirement age proposals', *Guardian*, 6 October 2009.

Criticisms have also been levelled at the party's efforts to court the 'green vote', not least with the adoption of the party's new green tree logo in preference to the long-serving blue torch. Cameron's decision to side with the Liberal Democrats and the Ghurkhas in their fight with the government clearly also played well with many voters, as has the party's admission that Margaret Thatcher was wrong when she asserted that there is 'no such thing as society'. The work that former party leader Iain Duncan Smith has done through his Centre for Social Justice (see Factfile) has offered the prospect of a more caring Conservative administration, finally shedding the 'nasty party' tag the Tories picked up in the 1980s.

Factfile Centre for Social Justice

- A right-of-centre think-tank that seeks to target poverty by forging links with voluntary groups and charitable institutions.
- Founded by former Conservative Party leader Iain Duncan Smith.
- Associated with two major reports: *Breakdown Britain* (2006), which outlined the problems facing the country; and *Breakthrough Britain* (2007), which suggested a range of remedies.

Though Cameron dropped references to 'progressive conservatism' in his 2009 address to the Conservative Party Conference, it is still unclear how he is going to reconcile his desire to adopt traditionally liberal positions on the environment and social welfare with pursuing the Thatcherite agenda of 'rolling back the frontiers of the state.' The kinds of changes envisaged can surely not be brought about entirely by voluntary groups and charitable institutions championed by many Conservatives. The economic crisis has seen the parties become more distinctive and coherent — as we will see elsewhere in this survey — but it is probably too early to speak of New Tories or a new Third Way, while the shape of what Cameron is trying to create is still so unclear. We may be witnessing the re-emergence of the more pragmatic one-nation Conservatism of the 1950s and 1960s as opposed to something truly new.

Will Cameron be able to carry the general public with him?

Public support for Cameron remained remarkably stable in the 18-month period between April 2008 and the end of September 2009; the eve of the autumn conference season (see Box 2.4). This was evidence, perhaps,

Box 2.4	Whatever happened to the 'Brown bounce'?			
'Which of these would make the best prime minister?'				
	Brown (%)	Cameron (%)	Clegg (%)	Don't know (%)
April 08	19	32	7	42
May 08	17	39	7	38
June 08	18	37	6	39
July 08	18	37	7	38
Aug 08	19	37	6	37
Sept 08	16	34	10	40
Oct 08	27	34	5	34
Nov 08	31	33	7	30
Dec 08	29	31	7	34
Jan 09	27	35	7	32
Feb 09	25	33	6	36
March 09	24	35	7	34
April 09	22	39	9	30
May 09	17	36	10	38
June 09	18	35	10	36
July 09	19	37	10	34
Aug 09	19	35	10	36
Sept 09	20	35	12	33

Source: YouGov *Daily Telegraph* political trends.

that Labour's tactic of branding Cameron and his Eton crowd as a bunch of Tory-toffs — first witnessed in the campaign against the Conservative candidate Edward Timpson at the 2008 Crewe and Nantwich by-election — had proven largely unsuccessful.

Such overt attempts to reignite some kind of political 'class war' ignore the fact that the class structure has changed significantly since the 1970s. Most of those who Labour is trying to fire-up are not prepared to write Cameron off purely on the basis of the family he was born into or the institutions at which he was educated. Such attacks also betrayed a desire to pass over inconvenient truths; not least, the fact that Blair's path to Oxford (via Fettes) was not in fact so very different from Cameron's (via Eton).

In truth, the only blip in support for a Cameron premiership was the fleeting 'Brown bounce' that came at the height of the economic crisis back in late 2008. As we predicted in our 2009 survey, however, this 'Brown bounce' proved to be little more than a 'dead-cat bounce', in economic parlance.

Such a consistent pattern of support for Cameron over Brown reflects a general and widespread dissatisfaction with New Labour's performance in office — the causes of which we will examine in other chapters of this survey. By the time of the YouGov *Daily Telegraph* tracking poll conducted at the end of September 2009, only 20% 'approved' of the government's record to-date; indeed, the figure had not topped the 22% mark at any point in the 9 months preceding the 2009 conference season.

What potential pitfalls will face Cameron if he becomes prime minister?

If we take nothing else from the New Labour experiment it is that even parties with large Commons majorities and a clear mandate for change can struggle to turn rhetoric into policy. Even the ban on fox hunting, now widely flouted, took close to 700 hours of parliamentary time and the use of the Parliament Act to bring it into law. New Labour's programme of constitutional reform — most notably Lords reform — quickly ran aground. Cameron, we should remember, may well not enjoy such large Commons majorities; the vagaries of demography and the electoral system meaning that the Conservatives might need to win the popular vote by ten percentage points nationally in order to get any kind of Commons majority (see 'UK Update', *Politics Review*, Vol. 18, No. 4).

It is clear that a good deal of thought has already gone into working out precisely how the Conservatives might learn lessons from Blair's early years in office (see Box 2.5). The way in which Cameron organises and makes use of the various institutions and individuals that comprise the core executive will clearly be key. It is now widely accepted that Blair's penchant for bilaterals and informal meetings ultimately proved counterproductive; not least as it served to marginalise and alienate those serving in cabinet. As James Forsyth noted in the *Spectator*, some see merit in the 'bee-hive' system employed in New Zealand whereby all ministers of cabinet rank work together in a single building — as opposed to being based in their departments where they can all too easily fall under the spell of senior civil servants and 'go native'. In this respect at least, the experience that both Cameron and Osborne had as special advisors in the last Conservative administration should hold them in good stead.

Box 2.5 **Avoiding the 'Blair-traps'**

Tony Blair is the model, but the model of what to avoid and not what to emulate. The Cameroons are confident they can learn from his mistakes. They point to Blair's failure to act decisively in his first few years in the job, the moment when he was strongest.

Source: J. Forsyth, 'Cameron has learned from Blair's failure to use his mandate and to command Whitehall', *Spectator*, 1 August 2009.

Conclusions

The economic crisis, which at first appeared to favour the former chancellor, Brown, and his party, ultimately played into the hands of the Conservatives, a party more comfortable with the language of spending cuts and public sector pay restraint. New Labour's hard-won reputation for economic competence was lost in a 6-month period during which even the former chancellor's achievements during a decade at No 11 were brought in to question. This economic context, allied to Cameron's rebranding of his party and the growing sense that it was 'time for a change' appeared to pave the way for a Conservative victory at the polls. However, being ready to win power is not the same as being ready to wield it. Though Cameron clearly has the intellectual ability to succeed in office he will need to address questions of 'delivery' during his first term, while his mandate is fresh and strong. Cameron must also find a way of reconciling his Thatcherite desire to 'roll back the frontiers of the state' with his oft-stated commitment to the environment and greater social justice for all (see Box 2.6).

Box 2.6 **For richer, for poorer**

David Cameron presented himself as a champion of the poor yesterday as he vowed to fight Britain's social ills more effectively than Labour. He brought the Conservative Party conference to its feet with an attack on Labour's 'big government', which he said had failed the most vulnerable. While maintaining that the Tories were still the party of enterprise he said that it now fell to them to fight for the poorest.

Source: P. Webster, 'For richer, for poorer', *The Times*, 9 October 2009.

Summary

- Although Cameron is well educated, his experience in government is limited to a spell as a special advisor during the last Conservative administration.
- Cameron's charisma and his ability to engage with the broader public have proven major electoral assets while in opposition and are likely to prove useful in government too.
- In many respects, both Cameron and his party find themselves in a position remarkably similar to that faced by Blair and New Labour ahead of the 1997 general election.
- If elected, Cameron will need to ensure that he makes the most of his party's mandate while it remains fresh and strong. This focus on 'delivery' will be particularly important if, as expected, the Conservatives only secure a small Commons majority.
- It is unclear how Cameron will manage to reconcile his commitment to the environment and greater social justice with his desire to pursue the Thatcherite goal of 'rolling back the frontiers of the state'.
- In short, it may be that Cameron is more ready to win power than to wield it.

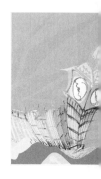

Chapter 3

MPs' expenses: an end to the gravy train?

Context

May 2009 saw the row over MPs' expenses — long smouldering — finally burst into flames with the *Daily Telegraph*'s publication in instalments of detailed expenses for virtually all frontbench and many backbench MPs. The impact of the *Telegraph*'s decision to publish was massive, both on those placed under close personal scrutiny and on public confidence in Parliament.

This chapter considers the fallout from the MPs' expenses scandal. In so doing it will address questions such as:

- What did the two main official reports into MPs' expenses uncover and what were their key recommendations?
- How effectively did the House of Commons authorities, the government and the main opposition parties respond to the crisis?
- Were MPs actually doing anything wrong?
- Who have been the major casualties of the scandal?
- Where now for MPs' expenses?

What did the two main official reports into MPs' expenses uncover and what were their key recommendations?

The first major review of some of the issues raised by the scandal came with the publication of a report by a panel chaired by former senior civil servant, Sir Thomas Legg, on 12 October 2009. Legg's remit had, in effect, been to conduct an audit of the expenses claimed by MPs in respect of their second homes. His decision to set levels of expenses that he considered reasonable and apply them retrospectively brought particular criticism from those MPs who had sought guidance and been given the 'all-clear' at the time they had submitted their original claims. There was even the suggestion that some of those ordered to pay back money might test the legality of this in the courts.

Despite opposition from the backbenches, however, Legg's recommendations received broad public support both from the prime minister, Gordon Brown, and the leader of the opposition, David Cameron: the latter went as far as to confirm that Conservative MPs who refused to repay the amounts would be barred from standing as Conservative candidates at the next general election.

The second and more far-reaching review of MPs' expenses came with the publication of the Twelfth Report of the Committee on Standards in Public Life — authored by that committee's chairman Sir Christopher Kelly — in

November 2009. Rather than considering the claims of individual MPs, Sir Christopher's report looked to the future by setting out seven principles of public life (see Box 3.1) and making 60 individually numbered recommendations; the 'highlights' are set out in Box 3.2.

How effectively did the House of Commons authorities, the government and the main opposition parties respond to the crisis?

The reaction of the Commons

There was widespread criticism of the way in which both MPs and the Commons authorities reacted to the crisis. As we saw in our 2009 survey, many MPs had originally hoped to keep details of their expenses secret by exempting themselves from the provisions of the Freedom of Information Act (2000) — the statute under which requests relating to MPs' expenses had first been tabled back in 2007. Although the 2007 Freedom of Information (Amendment) Bill was withdrawn before it could be rejected by the House of

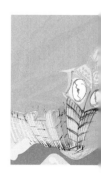

Lords, the failure of attempts to sidestep the freedom of information legislation in this way did little to win public support for the plight of MPs. The then speaker of the House of Commons, Michael Martin, faced particular criticism for his part in what appeared to be a deliberate attempt to block full disclosure. Martin failed in his attempt to block the implementation of the Information Tribunal's ruling though a judicial review. The leader of the House, Harriet Harman, also failed in her attempts to secure the passage of a Commons motion that would have had a similar effect to the original amendment.

Although the speaker argued that he had merely been discharging his duty to represent MPs in pursuing such action, his actions did little to enhance the reputation of, or public confidence in, the institution in which MPs were elected to serve. The same might also be said of the reaction of other senior figures in the Commons such as Harriet Harman, who was herself later caught up in the scandal as a result of the disclosure of her own expenses. The *coup de grace* came with the official publication of MPs' expenses for the period 2004–08 on Parliament's own website, the authorities having effectively censored (or 'redacted') whole sections of material that they felt might compromise the privacy or safety of members. For many commentators this was the final insult — with the full details already having been made available by the *Telegraph* following the earlier leak. The media reaction was, not surprisingly, savage, with many papers simply opting to publish pages from the official reports showing the blacked-out sections. Such coverage, at a time when public opinion had already moved decisively against MPs, further damaged the reputation of the Commons.

The reaction of the government and main opposition parties
'Heartfelt public statements and good intentions'
The leaders of the three main UK parties were a picture of humility in the face of the scandal. The Liberal Democrat leader, Nick Clegg, clearly had less to feel personally responsible for; his own party did not come under serious fire until nearly a week into the *Daily Telegraph*'s 'war' on expenses. Those Liberal Democrat MPs who did make it onto the inside pages were, on the whole, claiming hundreds of pounds as opposed to the thousands claimed by many Labour and Conservative MPs: Chris Huhne, for example, was 'exposed' as having claimed £119 for a Corby trouser-press. It was noticeable also that Liberal Democrats were able to avoid much of the scandal over mortgage interest relief and the so-called 'flipping' of second home status, an aspect of expenses that accounted for by far the biggest portion of the total Commons expenses bill.

Both Gordon Brown and David Cameron offered their apologies on behalf of those within their respective parliamentary parties who were said to have transgressed. Both leaders also confirmed that they would ensure that these MPs would repay monies claimed beyond the spirit as well as the letter of the rules, indicating that those refusing to repay monies would not be permitted to stand as official party candidates at the next general election. As we will see later on in this chapter, this pledge effectively ended the parliamentary careers of a number of senior members within each parliamentary party, as well as bringing the futures of many others into question.

The scandal also served to bring the broader issue of parliamentary and constitutional reform back onto the agenda, with several MPs taking the opportunity to make proposals that were frankly of only limited relevance to the issue at hand. Alan Johnson, for example, called for the introduction of alternative vote plus (AV+) in elections to the House of Commons, whereas some Conservatives favoured the introduction of US-style recalls as a means of removing incumbent MPs mid-term in cases of impropriety.

'Concrete changes'

The reaction to the *Daily Telegraph*'s publication of the leaked expenses details was every bit as 'knee-jerk' as efforts to address the issue over the previous 2 years had been ineffectual. As we have already noted in this chapter, former civil servant, Thomas Legg, was invited to conduct an audit of the expenses of individual MPs and the chairman of the Committee on Standards in Public Life, Sir Christopher Kelly, launched a 6-month investigation into

---

Box 3.3 **The Independent Parliamentary Standards Authority (IPSA)**

The Independent Parliamentary Standards Authority (IPSA) is a new and independent body created by the Parliamentary Standards Act (2009). The establishment of this new body will represent a break from old practices and put in place a new independent system for the payment of salaries and allowances for MPs. The IPSA is made up of four members and a chair, as below. Selection to the authority is on merit and by fair and open competition. The IPSA will:
- provide rigorous scrutiny and review of the allowances scheme for Members of Parliament
- prepare a code of conduct for MPs' financial interests
- support the commissioner for parliamentary investigations in cases where an MP is paid an allowance it is suspected he or she should not have been, or may have breached the code of conduct

IPSA chair (designate)
- Sir Ian Kennedy

IPSA board members (designate)
- Jackie Ballard
- Rt Hon Lord Justice Scott Baker
- Ken Olisa
- Professor Isobel Sharp

Source: IPSA's implementation website (www.parliamentarystandards.org.uk).

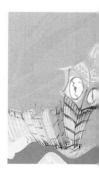

the issue of MPs' expenses and allowances that resulted in the publication of the committee's twelfth report in November 2009.

However, by far the most significant response to the crisis was the passage of the Parliamentary Standards Act (2009) into law in July 2009. This measure, rushed onto the statute books in a little under a month, established the new Independent Parliamentary Standards Authority (IPSA — see Box 3.3). This body, which takes on many of the roles of the discredited and now defunct Fees Office, is likely to be central to any attempt to make a better fist of the job of managing MPs' expenses and allowances going forward. Crucially, it will take a lead role in determining precisely how the recommendations outlined in Sir Christopher Kelly's report will be implemented.

Were MPs actually doing anything wrong?

The broader question of whether or not most MPs had actually done anything wrong was somewhat lost in the media frenzy surrounding claims for 'duck houses' and other such trivial issues (see Box 3.4).

First, one should remember that until recently it was not uncommon for public employees in various walks of life to receive generous relocation packages and allowances in recognition of the fact that they were in many cases agreeing

> **Box 3.4** **Some bizarre expenses claims**
>
> **Shalid Malik** (Labour, Dewsbury): £730 for a massage chair
>
> **Margaret Moran** (Labour, Luton South): £22,500 for dry-rot at her designated second home in Southampton
>
> **John Prescott** (Labour, Hull East): £312 for fitting mock-Tudor beams to his constituency home
>
> **Michael Ancram** (Conservative, Devizes): £99 for servicing the boiler that heated his swimming pool
>
> **David Heathcoat-Amory** (Conservative, Wells): £389 for horse manure
>
> **Douglas Hogg** (Conservative, Sleaford and North Hykeham): £2,200 for moat cleaning
>
> **Sir Michael Spicer** (Conservative, West Worcestershire): £620 for the installation of a chandelier; £5,650 for gardening, including the trimming of a hedge adjacent to a helipad
>
> **Sir Peter Viggers** (Conservative, Gosport): £1,645 for a 5ft floating duck house on his pond
>
> **Chris Huhne** (LibDem, Eastleigh): £119 for a Corby trouser press, £85 for mounting, framing and inscribing a photo of Chris Huhne
>
> Source: *Daily Telegraph*, May and June 2009.

to work for far lower salaries than they might reasonably have received in the private sector. The framework of MPs' allowances and expenses had, therefore, developed as a way of addressing the perceived shortfall in their basic salaries, with the alternative — a significant increase in those basic salaries — too controversial to consider. As the *Guardian* highlighted in an article on 17 November 2009, many other public employees receive a good deal more for their services than any MP: BBC broadcaster, Jonathan Ross, is said to enjoy a contract worth £18 million over 3 years; the heads of some newly nationalised banks have signed up for salaries in excess of £1.3 million per annum; and even DJ Chris Moyles is said to earn around ten times an MP's basic salary.

Second, most of those 'outed' in the *Daily Telegraph* had clearly remained within the letter, if not the spirit, of the rules established by the Commons authorities. Indeed, in many cases MPs who had approached the Fees Office uncertain as to whether or not certain claims were allowable had been given the 'all-clear'.

In line with their earlier pronouncements, the leaders of the major parties were quick to warn MPs within their party that they would face internal party sanctions if they did not agree to pay back the monies that Sir Thomas Legg judged unwarranted. There was, however, a clear sense of injustice in the minds of many that they should be blackmailed into paying back money claimed in good faith, within the rules as they stood at the time, simply on the say-so of a man who had chosen to apply far tougher limits retrospectively.

All of this is not to diminish the supposed offences of a handful of parliamentarians who may yet face criminal prosecution for fraud or false accounting, or those who are likely to face investigation by the Inland Revenue for failing to declare capital gains when selling their designated second homes. These are clearly more serious crimes and ones that, in some cases at least, appear to have been the product of premeditated planning and no little intelligence. For these MPs, the question posed ('Were MPs actually doing anything wrong?') must surely be answered in the affirmative, as they may in time be found to have done something that was not only morally questionable, but also illegal.

Who have been the major casualties of the scandal?

While it is simply not defensible that all those involved in the scandal could have been forced to give up their seats in the Commons, it is clear that the episode has cost some cabinet members their front bench positions and some rank-and-file MPs their entire political careers. In time, it might even result in one or two being imprisoned.

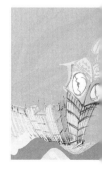

Stepping down from senior positions

By far the highest-profile casualty of the scandal was the Commons speaker, Michael Martin. Although the one-time Labour Member for Glasgow North East had faced criticism for his performance as speaker prior to the scandal, it was his handling of the expenses row that forced his departure on 21 June 2009. Martin's performance in respect of the crisis was criticised in two distinct ways: first, his failed efforts to prevent the publication of MPs' expenses through court action; and second, his reaction to the *Telegraph*'s revelations — criticising those MPs who had supported the paper's actions and launching an investigation into leaks as opposed to adopting the more conciliatory approach taken by the leaders of the main parties.

Other high-profile figures to fall on their swords in the wake of, or in anticipation of, revelations regarding their expenses were: the justice minister, Shalid Malik; the home secretary, Jacqui Smith; and the communities secretary, Hazel Blears. Although Smith and Blears might well have gone anyway in time — both had faced criticism in post and both were said to be dissatisfied with Gordon Brown's stewardship of the party — it was clearly the need to return to their constituencies and build bridges ahead of a likely general election that provided the final catalyst. For the Conservatives, the big-name casualty was Andrew MacKay, MP for Bracknell and David Cameron's policy aide, who, together with his wife (fellow MP Julie Kirkbride), was said to have claimed 98% of the maximum allowable in allowances by claiming for two homes.

Leaving Parliament to 'spend more time with their families'

While most of those resigning more senior positions did so with the intention of remaining in the Commons, at least at the outset, others chose or were forced to announce that they would not be standing at the next general election. Ian Gibson, for example, was told that he would not be allowed to represent the Labour Party in defence of his Norwich North seat. Although Gibson was initially said to be considering standing as an independent, he ultimately opted to resign, prompting the by-election that Labour lost on 23 July 2009 (see Chapter 1 of this survey). Two of those Conservative MPs whose expenses had prompted the greatest amusement in the press — Douglas Hogg ('moat cleaning') and Sir Peter Viggers ('duck house') — also announced their decision to step down at the end of the current term.

Facing criminal proceedings

While some of those caught up in the scandal lost their ministerial perks and others saw a premature end to their parliamentary careers, several were facing the prospect of legal action as 2009 drew to a close. On 23 November, the BBC reported that the Metropolitan Police had delivered files relating to four parliamentarians to the Crown Prosecution Service. The *Daily Telegraph* went further, by reprinting the details of six parliamentarians whose names it had disclosed the previous week and speculating that while only four files had been submitted up to that point, the files relating to the remaining two parliamentarians identified would be passed on to the CPS within weeks (see Box 3.5).

Box 3.5 **The prospect of legal action?**

Those facing prosecution are Labour MPs Elliot Morley, David Chaytor and Jim Devine, and peers Baroness Uddin, Lord Hanningfield and Lord Clarke of Hampstead. Four of the case files have been passed to the CPS, with a further two expected to follow within weeks.

Keir Starmer, the director of public prosecutions, is expected to decide whether to prosecute the politicians in the New Year, before a general election. Mr Starmer will determine whether the politicians face court on counts of fraud, which carries a maximum sentence of 10 years, or false accounting, for which the maximum penalty is 7 years. Police and criminal lawyers are confident that charges will be brought.

Source: *Daily Telegraph* (online), 23 November 2009.

'Casualties' in the broader sense?

By far the biggest casualty of the expenses row has been public confidence in the institution of Parliament. Although the massed ranks of independent candidates that looked likely back in the summer of 2009 will probably not materialise at the general election in 2010, it is likely that the more established minor parties will pick up support in some areas and that a number of those who 'fought on' in the face of the scandal will be ejected by their constituents at the ballot box.

Conclusions: where now for MPs' expenses?

At the height of the expenses scandal, when the leaders of the three main UK parties were caught full-square in the glare of the media's headlights, anything seemed possible: the speaker was forced to resign for the first time since 1695; MPs were to be stripped of their allowances and barred from holding second jobs; and recalls might even be introduced as a means of affording the general public the chance to remove errant MPs mid-term.

By November 2009, however, with the issue of MPs' expenses starting to fade in the public consciousness, much of what was mooted before the long summer recess appeared to have been forgotten. Gordon Brown refused to commit the government to implementing Sir Christopher Kelly's recommendations in full, arguing that it was for the newly-formed Independent Parliamentary Standards Authority (IPSA) to decide. Indeed, there was no mention of MPs' expenses in the Queen's Speech, despite the fact that Sir Christopher had personally briefed the press to confirm that 11 of the proposals outlined in his report would require primary legislation. A public row over the findings of

Sir Thomas Legg's report was also neatly side-stepped with the leaders of the main parties essentially forcing their MPs to pay back the money requested of them upon threat of de-selection. The notion that MPs, simply by paying back the sums claimed 'in error', could in effect draw a line under the matter appeared to fly in the face of all that had gone before. Yet by that stage even Julie Kirkbride (Conservative, Bromsgrove), who had earlier announced her intention to step down as MP at the next election, felt confident enough to put her head above the parapet and say that she was reconsidering her position and might yet stand — if the support was there at constituency level.

Quite where this leaves the issue of MPs' expenses is open to question. Although IPSA will in time, no doubt, consider Sir Christopher Kelly's recommendations and draft its statutory MPs' code of behaviour, it is hard to see how the matter will be laid to rest ahead of the next general election. Just as unclear is precisely what affect the scandal will have on voting patterns in that election — whether the successes of independents and minor parties such as the BNP and UKIP in last year's local elections and elections to the European Parliament will be translated into increased support at the next general election, or whether they will fall away badly again, just as they have in the past.

Summary

- The *Daily Telegraph*'s decision to 'serialise' leaked details of MPs' expenses between May and June 2009 pushed the issue to the top of the political agenda ahead of Parliament's summer recess.
- The leaders of the three main UK parties made full public apologies and promised to take a firm line with those within their parties who had overstepped the mark.
- The fallout from the scandal saw Michael Martin, the speaker of the House of Commons, and a number of ministers leave their posts.
- Several sitting MPs also announced their decision to step down at the time of the next general election, while others were barred from standing again by their parties.
- As the year drew to a close, six parliamentarians were said to be facing the prospect of criminal proceedings for fraud or false accounting.
- The crisis resulted in the passage of the Parliamentary Standards Act (2009) and with it the creation of an Independent Parliamentary Standards Authority (IPSA) that will produce the new statutory code of conduct for MPs.
- Two reports into MPs' expenses were published in 2009: Sir Thomas Legg's report took the form of an audit of the claims made by MPs between 2008 and 2009, whereas the twelfth report of the Committee on Standards in Public Life, authored by the Committee's chairman, Sir Christopher Kelly, made 60 separate proposals.
- The autumn Queen's Speech made no mention of MPs' expenses.

Chapter 4

UK political parties: how do they differ on policy?

Context

For a moment, late in 2008, it appeared that the deepening economic crisis might bring an end to the post-Thatcherite consensus and herald a return to a more adversarial style of party politics in the UK. For the Conservatives, David Cameron and George Osborne were urging massive spending cuts and cautioning against taking the nation further into deficit — while the prime minister, Gordon Brown, and his chancellor, Alistair Darling, were stressing the need to maintain levels of public expenditure at this key point in the economic cycle. However, in 2009, with the general election drawing closer, the gap between the two main parties appeared to narrow once more with differences again being measured more in terms of tone and emphasis as opposed to fundamental differences.

This chapter considers just how far the main UK political parties differ on policy ahead of the 2010 general election. In so doing it will address questions such as:
- How different were the policies being offered by the two main parties at the end of 2009?
- Have recent months witnessed a return to the adversarial politics of an earlier age, or are we seeing something entirely new?
- Where do the Liberal Democrats fit into the equation?
- How free will any government be to pursue its own policy agenda after the next general election?

How different were the policies being offered by the two main parties at the end of 2009?

The main battlefield in UK party politics in recent years has centred first on the core social policy issues of education and healthcare, and second on approaches to managing the UK economy. Party leaders who have sought to focus their party's campaigns on other policy areas — most recently the euro (William Hague, 2001) and immigration (Michael Howard, 2005) — have generally not fared well.

Social policy

The differences between the Labour and Conservative positions in most areas of social policy are still to be found more in tone and emphasis, than in principle. Indeed, the various policy priorities highlighted on the Conservative Party's website at the end of 2009 (see Box 4.1) could in most cases appear almost unedited on Labour's own site.

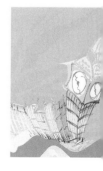

Box 4.1   Conservative policy, some headlines

1 Raising the bar, closing the gap
Our action plan to raise school standards

2 Power to the people
The decentralised energy revolution

3 Work for welfare
Real reform to help make British poverty history

4 Prisons with a purpose
Our sentencing and rehabilitation revolution to break the cycle of crime

5 A stronger society
Voluntary action in the twenty-first century

6 Delivering some of the best health in Europe
Outcomes not targets

7 Building skills
A training and apprenticeships revolution

8 The low carbon economy
Security, stability and green growth

9 Control shift
Returning power to local communities

10 Strong foundations
Building homes and communities

11 One world conservatism
A conservative agenda for international development

Source: www.conservatives.com

Education

The Labour Party has long since abandoned any plans to abolish the remaining state grammar schools, yet alone address the issue of private education. The Conservatives, for their part, appear equally happy with the status quo, focusing on 'shifting the balance of power away from government and towards parents' and 'encouraging smaller and more varied schools' as opposed to imposing a nationwide formula for secondary education. Both parties support the right of parents to establish new schools, both support the creation of new academies, and both agree on the need to improve school discipline and the quality of classroom teaching. The Conservatives' call to reduce bureaucracy and put power back into the hands of teachers is precisely what New Labour was calling for when in opposition back in 1996.

Healthcare

In the area of healthcare the gap between the main parties is also far less apparent than it used to be. The Labour Party is no longer committed to relying entirely on state provision, favouring public-private partnerships and the pooling of healthcare resources. The Conservatives also appear committed to the National Health Service, promising to provide 45,000 more single rooms in NHS wards and address the issue of drugs-pricing in order to ensure that new treatments are available to all, where they are shown to be clinically effective. Once again, the Conservatives are focusing on the need to remove top-heavy bureaucracy from the service and free-up NHS staff to do 'what they do best: providing top-quality care to patients'.

Economic policy

Economic policy was the area in which the two main parties were traditionally most clearly divided in their approach: with Labour said to support a more interventionist, 'big-government', tax-and-spend approach and the Conservatives favouring deregulation and a larger role for the market. New Labour's great achievement under Blair was to distance itself from these traditional positions by promising to stick to the Conservative's plans for taxation and spending. It was this commitment, alongside growing doubts over the Conservatives' ability to manage the economy following Black Wednesday in 1992, that allowed New Labour to develop a reputation for economic competence. It is no coincidence that in his efforts to restore public confidence in his own party's ability to manage the economy, David Cameron opted to do as Blair had done back in 1996 and commit his party to the plans established by the incumbent government.

However, it is in the area of economic policy that the parties have moved apart significantly since the end of 2008, a divergence brought about largely by the global credit crunch and the faltering fortunes of the UK economy.

The impact of the recession

The economic downturn prompted a significant divergence in the economic policies offered by the two main parties. The pattern was set early in the crisis, with the Conservatives opposing Brown's decision to nationalise Northern Rock. Thereafter the parties appeared to revert to more orthodox positions, with Labour opting to spend its way out of recession and the Conservatives urging caution and, crucially, withdrawing their pledge to hold to Labour's broad approach to running the economy once in office.

The Conservative Party's new position was clearly spelt out on its website:

> Gordon Brown has left Britain's economy ill-prepared for a downturn: he borrowed in a boom and left us with one of the biggest budget deficits in the advanced world; he stripped the Bank of England of its powers to supervise the City; he actively encouraged the risk-taking culture in our banks; and he claimed to have abolished boom and bust...Brown's economic mismanagement means that we can't offer big upfront tax cuts like some other countries.

This was a powerful attack on the prime minister and one that threatened to erode the political capital he had accrued during his decade as chancellor. Although few had expected the former chancellor to become a charismatic premier, most had trusted in his ability to manage the economy.

The Conservatives' prescription for the ailing UK economy was sweeping (see Box 4.2). They promised to restore the regulatory powers of the Bank of England and make significant cuts in government spending as a means of balancing the nation's books. In November 2009, David Cameron promised that an incoming Conservative government would deliver an emergency budget.

Box 4.2   Conservative economic proposals

- We will freeze council tax for 2 years by reducing wasteful spending on advertising and consultancy work in central government.
- We will introduce a £50 billion National Loan Guarantee Scheme and underwrite bank lending to businesses and get credit flowing again.
- We will provide tax cuts for new jobs with a £2.6 billion package of tax breaks to get people into work, funded by the money that would otherwise go on unemployment benefit.
- We will cut the main rate of corporation tax to 25p and the small companies rate to 20p, paid for by scrapping complex reliefs and allowances.
- We will give small- and medium-sized businesses a 6-month VAT holiday, funded by a 7.5% interest rate on delayed payments.
- We will cut National Insurance by 1% for 6 months for firms with fewer than five employees, paid for from the above changes to the company tax regime.
- We will abolish Stamp Duty for nine out of ten first-time buyers and raise the inheritance tax threshold to £1 million. Both of these changes will be funded by a flat-rate charge on non-domiciles.

To repair the broken economy in the long run, we need economic responsibility. That means:

- a responsible fiscal policy, bolstered by independent oversight
- a responsible financial policy, bolstered by a renewed role for the Bank of England
- a responsible attitude to economic development that fosters more balanced economic growth

Source: www.conservatives.com

In this area of policy at least then, clear fault-lines have emerged between the policies of the two main parties, with the Conservatives offering significant cuts in spending and a long-haul out of deficit and Labour promising to maintain public spending in most key areas.

Have recent months witnessed a return to the adversarial politics of an earlier age, or are we seeing something entirely new?

The age of adversarial politics saw the two main parties taking positions that were essentially ideological in nature. However, with the exception of economic policy, where there has been a real divergence in recent months, it is hard to make out such a clear division between the parties on most other key issues today. Certainly, in the major areas of healthcare and education — as we have seen — both the main parties appear to be offering the same solution, namely a partnership between the public and private sectors.

Moreover, critics have argued that the approach of both parties has become increasingly reactive and piecemeal. New Labour has long been criticised for being overly led by the media and — at least in Blair's first term in office — focus groups. In recent months, the Conservatives also appear to have taken a rather scatter-gun approach to announcing new proposals, with press releases on policy peppering the media with great regularity.

Although many of these proposals may eventually find their way into law, should the party be returned to office, some commentators have suggested that some policies have been put forward more for short-term media impact than as part of some joined-up programme for government. This was certainly a criticism levelled at the party's promise to raise the threshold for inheritance tax to £1 million — the pledge that was said to have contributed to Brown's decision not to call a snap election back in the autumn of 2007. Although such striking announcements have often served to erode Labour's support in the short term, they have also tied the Conservatives to policies that look increasingly untenable (see Box 4.3).

Box 4.3   Inheritance tax

Well, it looked like a clever idea at the time. Indeed it was a clever idea at the time. It was just over 2 years ago and the Tories smelt of panic as they gathered at their annual conference. Gordon Brown is on honeymoon with the voters. Labour has an election-winning advantage in the polls. Some members of the shadow cabinet seriously think David Cameron will no longer be Tory leader by Christmas.

All eyes are on his friend George Osborne. The young shadow chancellor gets to his feet, reaches into his hat and pulls out a pledge that only millionaires will pay inheritance tax under a Tory government. He claims that he can find the money by introducing a new levy on the 'non-doms'. His figures look a bit ropey, but the politics are sharp. A tax cut for British citizens paid for by unpopular wealthy foreigners: it's a great trick.

The cut to inheritance tax doesn't look so smart at all in the utterly changed political atmosphere of recessionary Britain. George Osborne's pledge has gone from being a lifesaver into an albatross around the necks of him and David Cameron.

Source: adapted from A. Rawnsley, 'Gordon Brown's favourite Conservative policy pledge', *Observer*, 29 November 2009.

A glance at the Conservatives' own website, where a total of 61 separate press releases were posted between 8 November and 1 December 2009, illustrates the problem. The party at times appears to be issuing proposals in all areas in the hope that some will appeal to voters and gain it support. A parallel can be drawn here with Cameron's efforts to find a label with which to encapsulate his personal take on conservatism. The media have dubbed Cameron's supporters 'New Tories', or more recently 'the Cameroons'. Cameron has also used a number of other phrases. Early in his leadership the Tory leader spoke of 'liberal Conservatism', later referring to his commitment to 'progressive Conservatism'. Former party leader Iain Duncan Smith's work with the Centre for Social Justice led some to use the phrase 'compassionate Conservatism', an echo of the kind of language used by the then presidential hopeful George W. Bush back in 2000. As with Conservative policy proposals this process has, at times, appeared to have more to do with finding a 'brand' that will fly with voters, than with setting out a coherent vision (see Box 4.4)

Box 4.4   Following rather than leading?

Between social science and politics falls the shadow of public opinion. Politics is often the mediation between fact and public sentiment. Bad politicians follow the focus groups and ignore inconvenient truths. Good politicians persuade the public of the necessary facts. Sensible scientists appreciate that this is a great and difficult skill: politics is an art that also deserves respect.

Source: P. Toynbee, 'Bad politicians are slave to public opinion. Good ones try to change it', *Guardian*, 27 November 2009.

What of Labour?

While one must necessarily make allowances for parties in opposition, those in government are expected to present a clearer vision of what they are doing and where policy is headed. In this respect Gordon Brown's administration has singularly failed to deliver.

In his book *Politics and Governance in the UK*, Michael Moran identifies three main ways in which the government's policy priorities can be established (see Box 4.5). Far from leading the process from the centre of the core executive, as one might have expected he would, Brown's premiership has been remarkably reactive in nature, with policy proposals often emerging either in response to events, or as a reaction to the policies proposed by the main opposition parties.

This observation is reflected in Brown's failure to establish a truly meaningful legislative programme during his time in office. Our verdict on the proposals

Box 4.5   Policy making

1 Business comes from within departments (through ministers/civil servants as a result of lobbying/research etc.)
2 Business comes from the core executive (cabinet, cabinet office, advisors etc.)
3 Business comes from fire-fighting (i.e. reactive as opposed to proactive)

Source: adapted from M. Moran, *Politics and Governance in the UK*, Palgrave Macmillan, 2005.

contained in the 2008 Queen's Speech, delivered in our 2009 survey, was fairly damning:

> While some of the bills outlined carried impressive titles, there was little that was truly ground-breaking... In some areas, the proposals simply restated or simplified what was already there, in other areas, proposals appeared to offer changes that would, in all probability, make little difference to most citizens' lives.

Such criticisms are equally applicable to the measures outlined a year later (see Box 4.6), with the added proviso that with only around 70 days of parliamentary business remaining before a general election must be called, few, if any, of the measures outlined are likely to pass into law. Such obvious limitations on the time available make some of the proposals contained in the 2009 Queen's Speech all the more unfathomable. What purpose could there be in offering a draft bill on Lords reform when New Labour has failed to deliver any real progress on this issue in over a decade? How would putting the government's existing commitment to end child poverty into law make it any more likely that the goal would be achieved? And why did the government feel the need to give legal force to the banning of cluster bombs, when it had already signed up to an international convention banning their future use? Ironically, perhaps, the things that could have been passed into law in the few weeks remaining (e.g. some of Sir Christopher Kelly's recommendations on MPs' expenses) were conspicuously absent from the speech.

| Box 4.6 | **The 2009 Queen's Speech** |

- Child Poverty Bill
- Bribery Bill
- Cluster Munitions (Prohibition) Bill
- Constitutional Reform and Governance Bill
- Fiscal Responsibility Bill
- Crime and Security Bill
- Digital Economy Bill
- Education and Families Bill
- Energy Bill
- Financial Services Bill
- Flood and Water Management Bill
- House of Lords Reform (Draft) Bill
- International Development (Draft) Bill
- Personal Care at Home Bill
- Equality Bill

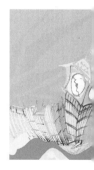

The pointlessness of the exercise was reflected in David Cameron's view, reported by the BBC, that the speech was the 'most divisive, short-termist, shamelessly self-serving' one 'in living memory'. It also explained the Liberal Democrat leader Nick Clegg's view that this Queen's Speech of 'fantasy bills' should simply have been delayed until after the general election.

Far from seeing a return to a previous age of ideologically-based, adversarial, conviction politics, therefore, British party politics in 2010 essentially remains an exercise in garnering votes, with the two main, catch-all parties arguing over the detail rather than the substance of policy.

Where do the Liberal Democrats fit into the equation?

The Liberal Democrats and their antecedents have traditionally occupied the centre ground in British party politics, with the Labour Party to the left on the political spectrum and the Tories to the right.

The decision of the Labour Party Conference to adopt its hard-left 1983 general election manifesto, which put the party into opposition for more than a decade, gave a boost to those at the centre. The Liberals, who had averaged only 9 seats in the 11 general elections between 1945 and 1979, had by that stage already benefited from the fresh impetus provided by the emergence of a new force in British politics, the Social Democratic Party (SDP). The union of the Liberals and the SDP, first in an electoral alliance in 1983 and 1987 and later as the Liberal Democrats, following the formal merger of the two parties in 1988, appeared to offer the prospect of genuine three-way party competition in Britain.

This has not proven to be the case, however. The genius of New Labour's electoral strategy was to fuse an acceptance of certain key elements of Thatcherite economic policy with the kind of radical constitutional reform agenda more traditionally associated with the Liberals. David Cameron's repositioning of the Conservatives since 2005 has had a similar effect in eroding support from the Liberal Democrats on the centre-right.

Table 4.1 Liberal Democrat performance at UK general elections

Year	Vote (%)	Seats
1983*	25.4	23
1987*	22.6	22
1992	17.8	20
1997	16.8	46
2001	18.3	52
2005	22.0	62

* SDP-Liberal Alliance

Source: adapted from E. Tetteh, *Election Statistics: UK 1918–2007*, House of Commons Research Paper 08/12.

UK Government & Politics

Although the Liberal Democrats retain a committed core following and benefit from significant levels of protest and tactical voting, the party Nick Clegg assumed control of back in 2007 has not really made significant progress in terms of electoral support since the SDP-Liberal Alliance first contested a general election back in 1983 (Table 4.1).

A change of tack?

It is largely an acceptance of this underlying truth that has resulted in Clegg's decision to adopt more radical policies and move the party away from the political centre, a shift that has led some to suggest that the Liberal Democrats and not Labour are now the most left-leaning mainstream political party in Britain. However, the reality is rather more complex than it might first appear, for while Clegg's approach in some areas appears to see the party adopting orthodox left-wing policies, in other areas it appears to be adopting a more traditional liberal (perhaps even neo-liberal) position. For example, while the Liberal Democrat leader promised over £20 billion in new spending on Liberal Democrat projects, such as support for nursing care, he planned to make an equivalent saving by shaving 3% off existing departmental budgets.

The party also offered the prospect of significant tax-cuts of between 4p and 6p in the pound, funded by efficiency savings and the closing of £5 billion of tax loopholes identified by the party's treasury spokesman Vince Cable. As Clegg himself explained to the *Guardian* back in September 2008, 'aspiring to hand back money to people from central government is impeccably liberal'. Clearly, all talk of tax cuts has had to be moderated in the wake of the economic crisis. However, before the crisis the Liberal Democrats were offering more radical economic policies at a time when others were refusing to commit.

In foreign policy also Clegg has offered something to those on the left (e.g. the possibility that the Liberal Democrats might opt not to upgrade Trident) as well as something for those on the right (e.g. the promise of a referendum on continued UK membership of the EU).

The Liberal Democrat approach is understandable. The party is fully aware of the need to maintain its broad appeal in order to attract disaffected voters from both of the two main parties: shift too far to the left and disaffected Tories might feel uncomfortable voting for the Liberal Democrats; lean too far to the right and alienate potential defectors from the Labour rank-and-file.

How free will any government be to pursue its own policy agenda after the next general election?

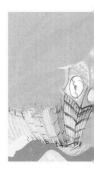

The ability of any incoming government to pursue its policy agenda from 2010 onwards will be limited first by the political realities of the situation it is likely to find itself in, and second by the economic realities that face the UK as the nation struggles to emerge from recession.

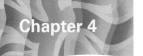

Political realities

It is extremely unlikely that the victorious party in 2010 will have anything more than a small Commons majority. Although the Conservatives have led Labour comfortably in opinion polls over the last 12 months, the electoral system and the existing constituency boundaries mean that they may well have to win by a margin of over 10% of the national popular vote in order to secure a working majority, and perhaps 5% even to be the biggest single party in a 'hung parliament'. Such analysis is far from fanciful; even in 2005 the Conservatives secured an average of 44,368 votes for each seat won (compared to Labour's 26,908).

If the Conservatives were in any doubt as to the scale of the challenge that faces them they need look no further than the kinds of gains in seats made by opposition parties at previous elections (see Table 4.2), with the Conservatives needing a gain of 128 seats in 2010 in order to secure a majority of one seat in the House of Commons.

Table 4.2 Seats won at recent general elections

Year	Labour	Conservative
1979	268 (−51)	339 (+63)
1983	209 (−59)	397 (+58)
1987	229 (+20)	375 (−22)
1992	271 (+42)	336 (−39)
1997	418 (+147)	165 (−171)
2001	412 (−6)	166 (+1)
2005	355 (−57)	198 (+32)

Source: based on data in E. Tetteh, *Election Statistics: UK 1918-2007*, House of Commons Research Paper 08/12.

Labour's chances of securing a sizeable majority also appear fairly small, with the best case scenario for the party appearing to be a repeat of 1992, when the party in government, John Major's Conservatives, clawed back a deficit in the polls to secure victory and a 21-seat Commons majority. A coalition government, often offered as the most likely outcome of a marginal result at a general election, is also unlikely since the most obvious coalition partner, the Liberal Democrats, is unlikely to want to commit to an exclusive relationship with either of the two main parties. It is quite possible, therefore, that the next government will have to work on a largely bipartisan, policy-by-policy basis.

Economic realities

The UK economy is unlikely to have recovered fully by May or June 2010, the likely date of the next general election. That — and the fact that any incoming government will have to pay off the accumulated national debt — means that any party in government will face serious constraints on what it can do.

Conclusions: what is the future of party policy in the UK?

While it is tempting to conclude that 2009 witnessed a return to a more orthodox, partisan, party politics in the UK, the evidence available simply does not support such a verdict. Although the economic downturn saw the two main parties taking a more adversarial approach when addressing issues of economic policy, there was still remarkably little to choose between them in most other areas of public policy. Indeed, what differences there are may ultimately count for very little, as the political and economic realities that will face the government elected in May or June 2010 will leave the victorious party with little or no room to manoeuvre.

Summary

- Recent years have seen a narrowing of the gap between the two main UK parties, a process that has led some to herald the 'end of ideology'.
- Under Tony Blair, New Labour became less committed to public-sector-only solutions and more open to market testing and public-private partnerships.
- Under David Cameron, the Conservatives have shed their image as the 'nasty' party and moderated their faith in 'the market' with renewed support for core public services such as the National Health Service.
- Although the economic downturn brought a return to a more familiar adversarial approach over economic policy, there were few significant differences between the two main parties in most areas of policy.
- It could be argued that the Liberal Democrats have in fact been offering more radical proposals than either of the two main parties, though the party has become increasingly difficult to locate on a traditional 'left–right', linear political spectrum.
- The party that wins the 2010 general election will have little room for manoeuvre on policy as a result of the political and economic context within which it will have to operate.

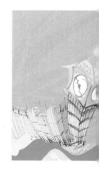

Chapter 5

Referendums: good or bad for UK democracy?

Context

Low turnout at recent general elections has prompted renewed interest in devices that might serve to address the challenge of political disengagement. A particular focus for debate in this context has been the question of whether or not the UK should make greater use of referendums as a means of resolving controversial issues and legitimising major constitutional changes.

This chapter considers whether the use of referendums in the UK since 1973 has served to enhance or undermine UK democracy. In so doing it will address questions such as:

- Why have there been calls for the wider use of referendums in recent years?
- How comfortably do referendums sit with the form of democracy traditionally practised in the UK?
- Has the UK experience of referendums thus far been a positive one?
- Have local referendums enhanced or undermined local democracy?
- Where to from here for referendums in the UK?

Why have there been calls for the wider use of referendums in recent years?

In 2009 UK-wide referendums were considered for two significant changes: first, the ratification of the Lisbon Treaty; and second, the question of electoral reform.

As we saw in our 2009 survey, the UK ratified the Lisbon Treaty without a referendum; the Labour government having determined that the new treaty did not warrant the kind of popular vote promised by all three major parties in respect of the EU Constitution it had replaced. However, while the confirmation of the UK's ratification of the treaty on 12 June 2008 should have put an end to calls for a nationwide referendum, this was not the case. Cameron's Conservatives offered the possibility of a retrospective UK referendum up until

Factfile — Referendum

- A vote on a single issue or policy proposal.
- Put to a public ballot by the government of the day.
- Generally framed in the form of a simple 'yes/no' question.
- Rarely used in the UK but employed more widely in countries such as Switzerland and in many US states.

the point at which the Czech Republic became the 27th and final EU member state to ratify the treaty on 3 November 2009.

Just as the Czech president was signing the Lisbon Treaty into law, ending any real chance of a UK referendum on the issue, the possibility of a nationwide ballot on another controversial issue moved a step closer. Though Labour had appeared to promise a referendum on electoral reform in its 1997 manifesto, little progress had been made towards that goal in the 13 years that followed. It was a surprise, therefore, that the closing months of 2009 saw serious discussion of whether or not the government might schedule a referendum on changing the system used in future elections to the Westminster Parliament on the same day as the 2010 general election. The question of precisely why such a referendum was being considered so late in the electoral cycle is addressed more directly in the UK Update section of *Politics Review*, Vol. 19, No. 3. Our focus here is more general: namely, why the offer of, and apparent support for, referendums has grown in the UK since the 1990s.

Why have referendums become more acceptable to a UK audience?

Three interlocking factors have fuelled support for the wider use of referendums in the UK in recent years: the participation crisis; New Labour's constitutional reform agenda; and the experience of such devices in operation, both in the UK and abroad.

The participation crisis

Referendums have been widely offered as one solution to the participation crisis identified both in the Power Report (2006) and in the media at large. Turnout at both the 2001 and 2005 general elections was significantly below the postwar average and referendums are commonly seen as a means by which decision making can at once be made more relevant to and closer to citizens. While some have argued that the decline in electoral participation has largely been cancelled out by a rise in non-electoral forms, most notably through increased pressure group activity, this is not in fact the case. Although certain forms of pressure group activity have been on the rise, there has been a decline in political participation in recent years — as demonstrated by Paul Whiteley in his articles in *Politics Review*, Vol. 19, Nos. 1 and 2.

Whether or not referendums will actually do a great deal to enhance political participation is another question entirely. Although referendums provide an additional opportunity to get involved, turnout and the quality of participation in such ballots is often disappointingly low, as we will see later in this chapter.

Constitutional reform

It has long been accepted that referendums might provide a way of legitimising major constitutional changes. A. V. Dicey referred to the referendum as a kind of 'people's veto' and modern UK leaders such as Tony Blair have largely accepted this argument: 'in the case of major constitutional change',

Blair remarked in 1995, 'there is clearly a case for that decision to be taken by the British people'. It is not surprising therefore that the programme of constitutional reform embarked upon by New Labour resulted in as many referendums being held in the party's first 2 years in office as had taken place in total up to that point.

The experience of referendums

The third and final reason why referendums have become more accepted in the UK relates to the way in which the UK's experience of such devices and awareness of how such devices are used in other countries has served to break down public mistrust of them.

The referendums held in the UK since 1997 have generally been well received. Though widely varying levels of turnout and the marginal 'Yes' vote in Wales in 1997 have prompted concern among political commentators, the broader public appear to have accepted the outcomes of such votes largely without question. The results of this shift have been twofold: first, the referendum as a device has become more acceptable to the public; and second, a precedent has been established in respect of future changes of a similar nature.

Greater awareness of the use of referendums outside the UK has contributed to the process by which referendums are now better understood and therefore more acceptable to UK voters. Coverage of referendums in other EU member states, particularly in respect of the ratification of major EU treaties, and awareness of the way in which citizens in many US states are able to influence

Table 5.1 Key US ballot initiatives in 2008

State	Proposal	Result
California, Florida, Arizona	Gay marriage ban	Passed
Nebraska	Ban on affirmative action in all state and local government programmes	Passed
Colorado	Ban on affirmative action in all state and local government programmes	Rejected
South Dakota	Ban on abortion except in cases of rape, incest, or where the mother's life is at risk	Rejected
Colorado	Human life to be declared as beginning with conception and abortion therefore to be classified as murder	Rejected
California	More humane treatment of farm animals	Passed
California	Financial incentives for the purchase of fuel efficient vehicles plus development of renewable energy technology	Rejected
Michigan	Allow for medical use of marijuana	Passed
Michigan	Allow stem cell research	Passed

Source: K. Moxon, 'Focus on...Referendums' *Politics Review*, Vol. 19, No. 3.

policy-making through devices such as referendums and citizen-initiated ballot initiatives (see Table 5.1) have even led political parties that have traditionally opposed the extension of direct democracy — most notably many Conservatives — to review their position.

How comfortably do referendums sit with the form of democracy traditionally practised in the UK?

Students of UK politics often reflect on the words of the one-time Labour prime minister, Clement Attlee, when assessing the merits of referendums in the UK. It seems appropriate, therefore, to use his words to provide a framework for our discussion.

'A device so alien to all our traditions'

Attlee's criticism can be interpreted in a number of ways. Taken literally, it was simply a statement of reality, i.e. the fact that referendums were not a feature of the UK political landscape in the 1940s, when Attlee was writing, or for that matter in the 1950s or 1960s. However, the comment also hints at a deeper meaning: the notion that the UK is essentially a 'representative' as opposed to a 'direct' democracy.

Under the representative model of democracy — sometimes referred to as the 'trustee' or 'Burkean' model — MPs are elected to represent the interests of constituents to the best of their ability. Crucially, however, those who represent us at Westminster are not simply delegates — issued with instructions outlining the way in which they are expected to act in the legislature. MPs are instead expected to apply their judgement to the questions of the day and to be prepared to go against the will of the people if they judge a particular course of action to be in the broader interests of those they serve. While individual MPs are ultimately held accountable to their constituents at election time, the majority party is generally seen as being free to use its mandate in seeking to bring into law the policies that it set out in its election manifesto; the doctrine of parliamentary sovereignty ensuring that no further authority need be sought from the citizenry before bringing such measures onto the statute books. Within a representative democracy, therefore, referendums would appear to be at best unnecessary and at worst counterproductive.

'A tool of dictators and demagogues'

Attlee's second criticism, like his first, was directly linked to the age in which he was writing. Whereas recent years have witnessed the rise of referendums as a means by which a government's mandate can be renewed or focused, Attlee would have been more familiar with the way in which totalitarian leaders such as Adolf Hitler had employed such devices as a means of legitimising courses of action that were not democratic. However, even in the modern era there is a case for arguing that referendums can result in a kind of tyranny of the majority, and that the majority in question may be ill-equipped to grasp precisely what is being asked of them.

Has the UK experience of referendums thus far been a positive one?

Although the public reaction to the increased use of referendums in recent years has been largely positive, the UK experience of referendums thus far has highlighted a number of problems. These are divided here into four broad categories: topic, wording, timing and turnout.

Topic

All nine ballots held thus far in the UK (see Table 5.2) have related directly to the distribution of power between supranational, national and subnational institutions. Whereas such changes inevitably fall within the definition of 'major constitutional reform' identified by Blair (see above), it is noteworthy that other equally significant changes, Lords reform for example, have not been legitimised by a public vote. The sense remains, therefore, that governments are inclined to offer referendums only on those issues where they have a direct interest in doing so, or where they are relatively certain of the outcome. This was certainly a criticism levelled at Harold Wilson's decision to go to the people in 1975 over continued membership of the EEC, an issue over which his Labour administration was deeply divided.

Table 5.2 Referendums sanctioned by the UK Parliament

Date	Who voted	Question (paraphrased)	Yes (%)	No (%)	Turnout (%)
1973 (March)	N. Ireland	Should Northern Ireland stay in the UK?	98.9	1.1	58.1
1975 (June)	UK	Should the UK stay in the EEC?	67.2	32.8	63.2
1979 (March)	Scotland	Should there be a Scottish Parliament?	51.6	48.4	63.8
1979 (March)	Wales	Should there be a Welsh Parliament?	20.3	79.7	58.3
1997 (Sep)	Scotland	Should there be a Scottish Parliament?	74.3	25.7	60.4
		...with tax-varying powers?	63.5	36.5	
1997 (Sep)	Wales	Should there be a Welsh Assembly?	50.3	49.7	50.1
1998 (May)	London	A London Mayor and London Assembly?	72.0	28.0	34.0
1998 (May)	N. Ireland	Approval for the Good Friday Agreement	71.1	28.9	81.0
2004 (Nov)	North East	A regional assembly for the North East?	22.0	78.0	48.0

Although Margaret Thatcher's reaction to that vote — declaring that referendums served only to 'sacrifice parliamentary sovereignty to political expediency' — is better applied to that one referendum than to referendums in general, the problem of precisely what kinds of issues require a referendum in the UK is a difficult one. Whereas most other countries have codified constitutions that clearly set out the circumstances in which a referendum must be held, or at least leave the decision to a supreme court, such decisions are left entirely to the whim of the party in office in the UK, as seen most recently with the decision not to offer a referendum in respect of the Lisbon Treaty.

Wording

Control of the precise form of words presented to the public in a referendum has also been a bone of contention in the past. The wording of the 1975 referendum on whether or not the UK should remain in the EEC was said to have been phrased in such as way as to encourage a positive response. Critics of referendums also criticise the way in which the precise details of the proposal are arrived at: for example, the decision to offer the Welsh an 'assembly' with 'secondary legislative' power in 1997, while at the same time offering the possibility of a Scottish 'parliament' with 'primary legislative' and 'tax-varying' powers.

Although the Electoral Commission was granted the authority to comment on the intelligibility of questions posed in all future referendums under the 2000 Political Parties, Elections and Referendums Act (PPERA) — see Box 5.1, p. 44 — the then deputy prime minister, John Prescott, was quick to confirm that the government (through its control of Parliament) retained the final say.

Timing

When considering the issue of timing, critics of referendums often highlight the possibility of ballots being scheduled close to events that might skew the result in favour of the outcome desired by the government of the day. However, the reality in recent years has been somewhat different: namely, that successive New Labour administrations have failed to schedule the referendums they have promised. For example, Tony Blair was clearly a supporter of UK entry into the euro, but the lack of support among the broader public meant that the referendum promised in the run-up to the 1997 general election did not materialise. While the need to meet the EU's 'convergence criteria' was initially offered in explanation of this failure to name a date for the ballot, there has been little progress in the last decade; even when the criteria were largely met, for a time, and other countries were allowed to work around the various tests and enter the eurozone.

Turnout

The problem with referendums is that while such devices are offered as a means of encouraging political participation and enhancing legitimacy, turnout at UK

> ### Box 5.1   Role of the Electoral Commission
>
> **Question assessment guidelines**
> 1 The question should prompt an immediate response.
> 2 Words and phrases used in the question should not have positive or negative connotations.
> 3 Words and phrases used in the question should not be intentionally leading.
> 4 Words and phrases used in the question should not be loaded.
> 5 The question should not contain 'jargon'.
> 6 The language used in the question should be consistent.
> 7 Words and phrases used in the question should reflect the language used and understood by the voter.
> 8 The question should not provide more information than is necessary to answer the question meaningfully.
> 9 The question should not be longer than necessary.
> 10 The question should be well structured.
>
> Source: The Electoral Commission.

referendums is often very low; bringing both of these stated goals into question. Though the latter problem can be addressed by the application of thresholds (i.e. by requiring a fixed percentage of the electorate to give a 'yes' vote, as opposed to a majority of those turning out), such artificial hurdles can create problems of their own, as seen in the Scottish devolution referendum in 1979. The reality is stark. Turnout at the nine referendums called by the Westminster Parliament has averaged just 57.5%; almost 2% below the mark set at the 2001 general election. While such low turnout at referendums is disappointing in itself, the problem is made worse still when the results in such referendums are marginal. The Welsh devolution referendum of September 1997 is a case in point; only 50.3% of the 50.1% who turned out favoured the establishment of the National Assembly of Wales.

Have local referendums enhanced or undermined local democracy?

Attention understandably often focuses on the nine referendums called by the Westminster Parliament between 1973 and 2004, but it would be wrong to ignore the increasing use of such devices at local level since the 1990s, both in approving structural changes to local government in some areas and in seeking to authorise policies such as the congestion charge.

Referendums on establishing directly elected mayors
The Greater London Authority, comprising a directly elected mayor of London and a 25-member assembly, was established following a referendum in 1998. Since then there have been more than 30 separate referendums on the question of whether or not to establish directly elected local mayors in places as distant as the Isle of White and Hartlepool.

The election of the Hartlepool FC mascot, H'Angus the Monkey (aka Stuart Drummond) as mayor in 2002 brought widespread criticism. How, it was argued, could an individual initially campaigning on a platform of giving free bananas to school children be placed in charge of a £106 million municipal budget? However, Drummond's performance in office and subsequent re-election in 2005 and 2009 led many to reconsider their position.

Although turnout at some of these local mayoral referendums has caused concern — ranging between 10% and 64% — the widespread use of such public polls has added to the sense that referendums are now part of the UK's democratic architecture.

Congestion charges

The congestion charge initiative originated with central government, but it was left largely to local authorities to adopt and implement. Whereas the first mayor of London, Ken Livingstone, used his considerable executive powers over London transport to introduce the charge, efforts to do so in Edinburgh (2005) and Manchester (2008) involved seeking public approval for the introduction of such charges through a local referendum (see Table 5.3).

Table 5.3 Congestion charge referendums

Year	Place	Turnout	'Yes'	'No'
2005	Edinburgh	61.7%	25.6%	74.4%
2008	Manchester	53.2%	21.2%	78.8%

While some regard the holding of such referendums and the resounding 'no' votes that resulted as a welcome exercise of 'pure democracy' or 'people power', others have been more cautious. In the case of Edinburgh, the cost of developing the proposals rejected in the referendum was estimated at £9 million — a considerable sum of money simply to write-off on the basis of what may well have been a knee-jerk reaction to the prospect of paying a new 'tax'. The rejection of charges in Manchester appeared to have been prompted by similar concerns (see Box 5.2). In both Edinburgh and Manchester the 'no' votes effectively prevented the improvements in transport infrastructure that those on all sides of the funding argument accepted were necessary. In the

Box 5.2 Ignoring the benefits

Ali Abbas, from Manchester Friends of the Earth group said 'I'm disappointed at a missed opportunity. It was a great chance for us to make a huge improvement to our transport and to help to tackle greenhouse emissions. When we asked people why they wouldn't vote for it they told us that 'we won't vote for it because the transport is so bad'. But our argument was 'if you vote for it, the transport will get better'.

Source: 'C-charge: a resounding 'NO', *Manchester Evening News*, 12 December 2008.

case of Manchester the 'no' vote was particularly significant as the transport secretary, Geoff Hoon, had already conceded that there was no 'plan B' for improving transport in the city. As Lord Peter Smith, chairman of the Greater Manchester Authorities, commented to the *Manchester Evening News*, the result was 'very clear…this is not just a vote no for congestion charging, it is a vote no to improvements on the trams, railways and buses and there will now be no improvements'.

Conclusions: where to from here for referendums in the UK?

Despite the promise of a number of referendums in recent years, it remains the case that the vast majority of English people under the age of 50 have never had the opportunity to vote in a major UK referendum. The nine referendums called by the Westminster Parliament since 1973 have focused on an extraordinarily narrow range of issues. The way in which such ballots have been conducted and the low levels of turnout witnessed have raised issues of legitimacy that go beyond simply questioning whether or not such devices are compatible with our representative democracy.

However, while there is no great clamour for the adoption of the kind of process seen in many US states and in some European countries, public support for the wider use of referendums appears to be increasing. This greater public acceptance, allied to the prospect of further constitutional reform whichever party wins the next general election, makes it likely that such devices will be used a good deal more in the coming years.

Summary
- The UK has seen a growth in support for the use of referendums in recent years.
- This support has resulted from three key factors: widespread concern over declining levels of political participation; the constitutional nature of many of the measures proposed by New Labour its victory at the 1997 general election; a positive reaction to the use of referendums, both domestically and abroad.
- Although Clement Attlee's reservations regarding the use of referendums in the UK have weakened in relevance over time, such devices may still pose a threat to the style of representative democracy practised in the UK.
- Critics argue that voters do not always understand precisely what is being offered and are too inclined to deliver short-term, knee-jerk verdicts on proposals that might bring significant — if less immediately apparent — long-term benefits.
- Low turnout at both national and local referendums in the UK raises questions of legitimacy — as do issues relating to the precise circumstances in which referendums might be required, how referendum questions are framed, and control over the timing of such ballots.
- The widespread acceptance of referendums means that such devices are now an established part of the UK's democratic architecture.

Chapter 6

New Labour and constitutional reform: promise unfulfilled?

Context

As we head towards a 2010 general election — and what may well prove to be the end of New Labour's 13 years in office — it seems appropriate to consider and offer a tentative assessment of the party's achievements in the area of constitutional reform.

This chapter considers precisely how far the Blair and Brown administrations have gone towards delivering the ambitious proposals set out in their 1997 general election manifesto. In so doing it will address questions such as:

- Was Brown offering anything that was genuinely new in 2009?
- What had New Labour set out to achieve back in 1997?
- What have been the success stories of New Labour's constitutional reform programme?
- In what areas has actual policy failed to live up to the rhetoric — and why?
- Where now for constitutional reform?

Was Brown offering anything that was genuinely new in 2009?

Gordon Brown's accession as Labour leader and prime minister in 2007 raised hopes of a fresh impetus for New Labour's stalled programme of constitutional reform, but the *Governance of Britain* Green Paper (2007) and the subsequent Constitutional Renewal Bill (2008) led many to conclude that major changes would have to wait until after the next general election at the earliest.

It was something of a surprise, therefore, that the Labour leader used his speech setting out the government's response to the scandal over MPs' expenses on 10 June 2009 to announce that the Democratic Renewal Council — Brown's cabinet committee on constitutional reform — had approved a number of 'new' constitutional proposals (see Box 6.1).

While there is clearly considerable public support for many of the measures Brown proposed (see 'UK Update', *Politics Review*, Vol. 19, No. 1), the truth is that few if any of the proposals outlined by the prime minister are genuinely new and none are likely to be realised ahead of the 2010 general election. This reality was reflected in the modest scope of the Constitutional Reform and Governance Bill introduced a day before Parliament rose in July

2009; a bill that was, in effect, little more than a watered down version of the Constitutional Renewal Bill that had been met with such derision a year earlier.

| Box 6.1 | Brown's June 2009 constitutional reform proposals |

1 The completion of Lords reform
2 A debate over a new bill of rights and a written (i.e. codified) constitution
3 Further devolution and an effort to engage people in their local communities
4 Electoral reform
5 Increasing public engagement in politics

Source: *Monitor*, Issue 43, The Constitution Unit, September 2009.

The limited scope of what has been achieved (or for that matter proposed) under Brown means that our assessment of New Labour's record on constitutional reform needs to focus on what was established under Tony Blair, the man he succeeded at No 10.

What had New Labour set out to achieve back in 1997?

The list of proposals that New Labour set out in its 1997 general election manifesto was, by any standards ambitious, both in scope and in depth (see Box 6.2). Eighteen years in opposition had afforded the party ample time to establish an agenda for action and groups such as Charter 88 had clearly influenced the thinking of many of the party's leading lights.

Most of the proposals, however, with the possible exception of the offer of a 'human rights act' and a bipartisan approach to the Northern Ireland peace process — were based more on the Labour Party's experience in office and opposition, than on political principle.

The proposals on Lords reform and electoral reform can certainly be seen in this light. The presence of over 750 hereditary peers in the unreformed Lords had afforded the Conservative Party an in-built majority. Put simply, the rarely-present Tory 'backwoodsmen' could normally be relied upon to attend Parliament when needed to defeat radical proposals. This fact — not withstanding the inequity inherent in the hereditary system — was alone sufficient to merit Lords reform in the eyes of many of those within the Labour Party.

The first-past-the-post electoral system used in elections to the Westminster Parliament had been a similar source of angst for New Labour while in opposition. A fourth consecutive general election defeat in 1992 had led some leading commentators to question whether or not the Labour Party would ever be able to win again under the system in place — so clearly was it said to favour the Conservatives. It was during these bleak years that many within the party became wedded to the idea of electoral reform.

Box 6.2 **Labour's 1997 manifesto pledges**

Lords reform
- 'Remove the right of hereditary peers to sit and vote' in the Lords.
- Reform the Lords to make it more 'democratic and representative'.

Commons reform
- Establish an investigation into House procedures.
- Make Prime Minister's Questions 'more effective'.
- Regulate party funding.
- Offer a referendum on electoral reform once an independent commission has made its recommendations.

Open government
- Introduce a 'Freedom of Information Act'.
- Establish an independent 'National Statistical Service'.

Devolution
- Hold Scottish and Welsh devolution referendums by the autumn of 1997 (with no threshold).
- Offer the Scots a Parliament with both primary legislative powers and 'tax varying powers'.
- Offer the Welsh an Assembly with 'secondary legislative powers'.

Good local government
- Give greater power to local councils.
- Provide for a proportion of councillors to be 'elected annually' to provide 'greater accountability'.
- Introduce elected mayors with 'executive powers' in some cities.
- Establish a new 'strategic authority' and mayor for London.
- Hold referendums, 'region by region', on the creation of directly elected regional governments.

Real Rights For Citizens
- Incorporate the European Convention on Human Rights (ECHR) into UK law as a 'floor' not a 'ceiling' for the rights of UK citizens.
- Establish legally enforceable rights for the disabled.

Northern Ireland
- Build on the Anglo-Irish Agreement, the Downing Street Declaration and the Framework Document to move towards the establishment of a devolved legislative body.

Source: 'New Labour: because Britain deserves better', 1997 Labour Party Manifesto, pp. 32–35.

The various other Commons reforms and the offer of a Freedom of Information Act should be seen in the context of events around the time of the 1997 general election; in particular the allegations of sleaze and corruption that had dogged the final years of John Major's Conservative administration. The devolution proposals were unfinished business for Labour, following the 'failed' referendums of 1979. The desire to empower local government reflected the way in which many Labour-controlled local councils felt they had suffered at the hands of the Conservative government in power at Westminster; not least with the abolition of the Greater London Council and the Metropolitan Counties in 1986 and the imposition of rate-capping.

What have been the success stories of New Labour's constitutional reform programme?

Although unqualified successes and unmitigated disasters are relatively rare in modern politics, it is clear that some aspects of New Labour's programme of constitutional reform have gone better than others, specifically: devolution; the Human Rights Act (1998) and Freedom of Information Act (2000); and judicial reform.

Devolution: a success story?

The reaction to devolution among the populations of Scotland and Wales has been a largely positive one — as we shall see elsewhere in this survey (Chapter 8). This is hardly surprising. While the cost of establishing and maintaining devolved institutions has been considerable, devolved government has brought tangible benefits to the people of each nation.

North of the border, the Scottish Parliament has offered free nursing care to the elderly, has refrained from introducing university top-up fees or establishing foundation hospitals, and has lifted toll charges on the Skye bridge, a *cause célèbre* of Scottish pressure group activity for more than a decade from the mid-1990s.

Despite possessing more limited powers, the Welsh Assembly has also been able to adopt popular, radical policies in a number of areas — for example, with the removal of prescription charges. Indeed, by 2011 it is likely that England will be the only one of the home nations where prescription charges still apply.

Though the West Lothian Question (see p. 73) and the broader question of precisely where the process is 'going' remain unanswered, devolution is widely seen as a New Labour success story; not least because it took the momentum out of the nationalists' campaigns for full independence.

The Human Rights Act and Freedom of Information Act: a new rights culture?

In passing the Human Rights Act (HRA) in 1998, Labour fulfilled its 1997 manifesto commitment to incorporate the European Convention on Human Rights (ECHR) into UK law. In a similar vein, the passage of the Freedom of Information Act (FOI) in 2000 sought to deliver on the promise to provide more transparent government.

Both measures have attracted criticism — the HRA in its application and the FOI for its modest scope — but they may both come to be seen as historically significant. Though the first attempts at reform in a given area rarely meet with universal approval, they often come to be seen as significant landmarks on the road to something more meaningful and lasting; witness the status now afforded to the Great Reform Act of 1832 — in itself a rather modest reform.

It is worth remembering that Labour's efforts to advance its reform agenda in these areas have been hindered by circumstance. The attacks of 9/11 and 7/7 fundamentally changed the domestic security landscape, forcing the passage of new anti-terror legislation and with it the derogation of some of the ECHR's provisions — while at the same time limiting the government's willingness to extend the terms of the FOI.

Against that backdrop it is perhaps all the more remarkable that none of the major UK parties is talking about simply 'turning the clock back' in these areas. Instead, Brown is said to be considering extending the scope of the FOI and all three parties are talking either of enhancing and re-working the HRA or replacing it with a more formal bill of rights; perhaps incorporating an outline of civic responsibilities and duties alongside those rights identified.

Judicial reform: a more independent and effective judiciary?
The area of judicial reform, largely unheralded in New Labour's 1997 manifesto, has perhaps seen the most marked changes in recent years. Proposals originally unveiled in 2003 gave rise to the Constitutional Reform Act (CRA) in 2005 which in turn led to the establishment of a new independent Judicial Appointments Commission (JAC), a re-working and downsizing of the role of Lord Chancellor, the emergence of a new Justice Ministry and the creation of a new UK Supreme Court located in Middlesex Guildhall.

The last of these developments may well, in time, prove to be the most significant. The new court, which opened for business at the start of the legal year on 1 October 2009, could yet take on a status and significance wholly unforeseen at the time the CRA passed into statute.

In what areas has actual policy failed to live up to the rhetoric — and why?

While New Labour has made significant progress in some aspects of constitutional reform, the steps taken in other areas (namely Lords reform, Commons reform and electoral reform) have been somewhat smaller and more tentative.

Lords reform: a false start?
New Labour's manifesto commitment to remove the right of hereditary peers to sit and vote in the Lords was largely fulfilled with the passage of the House of Lords Act (1998). Although 92 former hereditaries remain, under the terms of the Weatherill Amendment, this reform has contributed to a significant shift

in the party balance within the Lords — effectively wiping out the in-built Tory majority that had existed in the Lords prior to the Act coming into force in 1999 (see Table 6.1).

Table 6.1 The composition of the Lords

Affiliation	1999	2009
Conservative	471	192
Labour	179	213
Liberal Democrat	72	71
Crossbench	353	183
Other (including bishops)	219	48

Though this was envisaged as just the first phase in a programme of reform that would see the Lords emerge as a more 'democratic and representative' upper chamber, it has since proven impossible to reach a consensus on precisely what the second phase of Lords reform should entail. The result of this impasse is that the UK is, in effect, still operating under the transitional arrangements established more than a decade ago.

The failure to complete the reform of the Lords is often used as evidence of New Labour's broader failure to deliver on constitutional reform since 1997. Commons majorities of 178 (after 1997) and 166 (after 2001) should have afforded Blair and New Labour the freedom to shape the upper chamber in the style desired. Their failure to do so stems first from the fact that there was never any clear idea as to precisely what was desired, and second from the fact that the part-reformed chamber has in fact performed remarkably well.

While Lords reform must therefore be seen as a failure when viewed purely in terms of New Labour's stated aims — witness also the shambolic failure of the People's Peers initiative and the shame of the 'cash for peerages' investigation — the part-reformed Lords could just as easily be seen as one of the success stories of New Labour's programme of constitutional reform.

Commons reform: ineffective and unfinished?

Labour's 1997 manifesto offered a comprehensive review of Commons procedures, a re-working of Prime Minister's Questions (PMQs) and proper regulation of party funding.

The party certainly delivered on its promise to change the procedures surrounding PMQs. The two 15-minute sessions on Tuesdays and Thursdays became a single 30-minute slot on Wednesdays and the convoluted conventions relating to the way in which questions had to be addressed to the prime minister were streamlined (see Box 6.3).

Though such changes were aimed at making PMQs a more meaningful forum for holding the prime minister to account, it is still widely seen more as theatre than serious politics. In addition, some parliamentarians have mourned the loss of the shorter, twice-weekly sessions; if only because they required the prime minister to attend the Commons on at least two occasions each week.

New Labour's attempts to regulate party funding have proven rather more problematic than its tweaking of PMQs. While its Political Parties Elections and Referendums Act (PPER) in 2000 required all major donations to political parties to be recorded and publicly declared, the Labour party itself side-stepped the regulations by encouraging potential backers to offer long-term loans at preferential rates, as opposed to straight donations. Though the police investigation into the allegation that such loans were linked to the granting of peerages did not ultimately result in criminal prosecutions under the Honours (Prevention of Abuses) Act of 1925, the perception remained that New Labour had sought to conceal the scale and source of monies it had received. The emergence of the MPs' expenses scandal, coming so hot on the heels of the cash for peerages scandal, only served to add to the sense that Labour had fallen some way short of delivering on its 1997 pledge to 'clean up politics'.

While there have been some significant, if relatively small, changes in Commons procedures (e.g. changes in working hours and sittings) the big changes that many hoped would emerge following the work of the Select Committee on the Modernisation of the House of Commons have in many cases failed to materialise. Though both Blair and Brown have submitted themselves to 6-monthly scrutiny at the hands of the Liaison Committee, the powers of select committees in general have not been greatly enhanced in the way envisaged in the Newton Report (2001) and many subsequent studies. Indeed, in October 2009 the children's secretary, Ed Balls, raised the ire of the Children, Schools and Family Select Committee by ignoring its recommendation and appointing Maggie Atkinson to the post of children's commissioner.

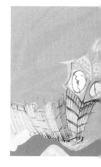

The enhanced parliamentary scrutiny of the executive trailed in the *Governance of Britain* Green Paper has simply not been carried through into statute.

Electoral reform: a failure to deliver?

Though Labour's manifestos in 2001 and 2005 confirmed that a referendum on electoral reform would take place only once a decision to change the system used in elections to the Westminster Parliament had been made, the party's 1997 manifesto had been unequivocal (see Box 6.4); most if not all of those voting for the party would surely have assumed both that a referendum would happen and that it would take place sooner rather than later.

Box 6.4 **Labour on electoral reform**

Labour's 1997 manifesto
We are committed to a referendum on the voting system for the House of Commons. An independent commission on voting systems will be appointed early to recommend a proportional alternative to the first-past-the-post system.

Labour's 2001 manifesto
We will review the experience of the new systems and the Jenkins Report to assess whether changes might be made to the electoral system for the House of Commons. A referendum remains the right way to agree any change for Westminster.

Labour's 2005 manifesto
Labour remains committed to reviewing the experience of the new electoral systems — introduced for the devolved administrations, the European Parliament and the London Assembly. A referendum remains the right way to agree any change for Westminster.

In the event — and despite the Jenkins' Commission recommending a far less controversial system (AV+) than some had expected the Liberal Democrat peer to favour — electoral reform for elections to the Westminster Parliament has simply not been on Labour's agenda for more than a decade.

While the Labour administrations have overseen the introduction of alternative electoral systems in other arenas (see Box 6.5), such systems have normally been adopted with specific goals in mind. Examples are: the party list system, to fall into line with elections to the European Parliament in other EU member states; and the single transferable vote, to address concerns about the impact of sectarianism on elections in Northern Ireland. Some even saw the adoption of the supplementary vote system in elections to the post of London mayor as a cynical move designed to maximise Labour's own chances of success.

The operation of all three systems — along with the additional member system in elections to the Scottish Parliament, the Welsh Assembly and the London

Assembly — has provided ample evidence as to how electoral reform at a national level might affect governance in the UK. However, despite Labour's promise to 'review' and build upon the 'experience' under such systems, more than a decade has now passed without any real progress on the question of reforming the system used in UK general elections.

Box 6.5 UK electoral systems

First-past-the-post: elections to the Westminster Parliament and most local elections in England and Wales.

Supplementary vote: elections for London mayor and other directly elected mayors.

Closed regional party list: British elections to the European Parliament (Northern Ireland uses single transferable vote).

Single transferable vote: Assembly, local and European elections in Northern Ireland and Scottish local elections (since 2007).

Additional member system: elections to the Scottish Parliament, the Welsh Assembly and the Greater London Assembly.

To a degree it is always the case that parties who favour electoral reform during lengthy spells in opposition, come to see the merits of the simple plurality system once they are returned to office. This observation has certainly been true of New Labour's spell in office between 1997 and 2009. Indeed, it is only now that electoral defeat appears likely that electoral reform is back on the agenda, with some Labour insiders arguing that a referendum on reform should be scheduled to coincide with the 2010 general election.

Local government: a democratic deficit?

Labour's 1997 manifesto committed the party to reinvigorate local government, rendering it both more independent of central government and more accountable to those it serves. The party pledged to move power from the centre out, employing the principle of subsidiarity. In a move designed to reverse Margaret Thatcher's abolition of the Greater London Council in 1986, Labour offered a new strategic authority and directly elected mayor for the capital — as well as the prospect of directly elected mayors in other parts of the UK. By far the most far-reaching of New Labour's promises, however, was its commitment to creating a new tier of directly elected regional government, legitimised by referendums that would be held 'region by region'.

While the last 13 years have indeed witnessed the creation of devolved government in London and other directly elected mayors outside of the capital — most notably with the installation of the Hartlepool FC mascot H'Angus the Monkey (aka Stuart Drummond) as mayor of Hartlepool in 2002 — Labour's plans for local and elected regional government beyond that have fallen flat. When the first referendum on the establishment of an

English regional assembly finally came in 2004, it was held not in the West Midlands or the South West (where support might have been a good deal stronger) but in the North East; a region long-associated with low electoral turnout. Though the cabinet had finally bowed to John Prescott's demand for a referendum to be held, the comprehensive 'no' vote delivered by the people of the North East effectively put an end to Labour's plans for directly elected regional government in England. Some even suggested that Labour's decision to hold the poll in the North East with the offer of such a limited, yet potentially costly, assembly was purposely designed to result in such an outcome; Labour had, in effect, offered the people least likely to turn out and vote 'yes', the thing that they least wanted.

The mothballing of New Labour's plans for directly elected regional government has not, of course, resulted in any slowing in the growth of unelected regional government. Indeed, Labour has presided over the creation of a regional quangocracy of quite immense proportions over the course of its 13 years in office. Far from making local government more relevant and accountable to the people it serves — the aim set out in 1997 — Labour has in fact delivered quite the opposite.

Conclusions: where now for constitutional reform?

New Labour's 1997 manifesto offered an impressive mission statement (see Box 6.6) as well as establishing an incredibly ambitious — perhaps too ambitious — set of objectives in the area of constitutional reform.

Box 6.6	Where did it all go wrong?

Our aim is no less than to set British political life on a course for the future. People are cynical about politics and distrustful of political promises... What follows is not the politics of 100 days that dazzles for a time, then fizzles out... We will clean up politics, decentralise political power throughout the United Kingdom and put the funding of political parties on a proper and accountable basis.

Source: taken from Tony Blair's introduction to 'New Labour: because Britain deserves better', the 1997 Labour Party Manifesto, pp. 1–5.

Though the party's success in delivering on its promises in this area of policy has clearly been mixed, one should remember that the significance of such constitutional changes — both in terms of their intrinsic merit and their place along the road to better governance — may only become apparent with the benefit of hindsight. While it is therefore tempting to write-off New Labour's programme of constitutional reform as a rather piecemeal and incomplete attack on the problems the party identified during its 18 years in opposition, it is likely that some or all of the reforms will ultimately come to be seen in a better light.

What is clear, however, is that New Labour could have made a good deal more of the enormous Commons majorities and popular mandates secured at the 1997 and 2001 general elections. This is a lesson that has clearly not been lost on David Cameron's Conservatives, as we see elsewhere in this survey.

Summary

- New Labour's 1997 manifesto set out an incredibly ambitious programme of proposals in the area of constitutional reform.
- The massive Commons majorities and popular mandates secured in 1997 and 2001 presented the party with an opportunity to do largely as it pleased.
- In some areas (e.g. devolution, judicial reform, the Human Rights Act) progress has been more far-reaching and more rapid than in others (e.g. Lords reform, electoral reform and elected regional government).
- Labour's efforts to establish a rights-culture have been hindered by events such as 9/11 and 7/7.
- Though many initiatives appear incomplete, we should recognise that incremental change is in fact the norm in the area of constitutional reform; New Labour's legacy is to have set the ball rolling.

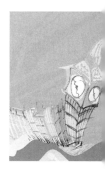

Chapter 7

'Goodbye' Human Rights Act, 'hello' Bill of Rights?

Context

October 2010 would mark the tenth anniversary of the Human Rights Act (HRA) coming into force, yet this landmark may well prove to be a bridge too far for a measure that has been subject to sustained criticism in recent years. David Cameron's Conservatives, if elected, are committed to replacing the HRA with a British Bill of Rights. Labour, the architects of the HRA, favour developing what is there already into a more coherent bill of rights and responsibilities.

This chapter revisits and reassesses the verdict we delivered on the HRA in our 2007 *Annual Survey*, as well as looking forward to what might happen in this area of policy following the 2010 general election. In so doing it will address questions such as:

- What did the two main UK parties propose in respect of the HRA in 2009?
- Are such proposals warranted?
- What problems might such proposals present?
- Is it possible to have a meaningful Bill of Rights in the absence of a properly codified and entrenched constitution?

What did the two main UK parties propose in respect of the HRA in 2009?

As is the case in many other areas of policy, the Conservative and Labour positions on the HRA do not appear to differ greatly (see Box 7.1). While the Conservatives' commitment to replace the Act would offer more encouragement to its critics than Labour's offer of consultation, both parties appear to accept the basic premise that something must be done in order to address public concern over the application of the HRA.

Box 7.1	Conservative and Labour positions on the HRA

Labour: 'A green paper to examine the case for developing a Bill of Rights and Responsibilities. A dialogue with the British public about how we might develop and articulate an inclusive view of our shared values.'

Conservative: 'Replace the Human Rights Act, which has undermined the government's ability to deal with crime and terrorism, with a British Bill of Rights.

Source: Conservative Party and Labour Party websites, December 2009

Labour's approach

As we noted in our 2007 *Annual Survey*, 'one would hardly expect the Labour government to abandon the Human Rights Act — given that it was they that introduced the measure in 1998'. However, the declining public confidence in the Act and the popular appeal of the Conservatives' promise to scrap it and offer a uniquely British replacement has forced the government into rethinking its strategy over the last 3 years, to the disappointment of many of those on the liberal-left.

Back in 2006, the then Lord Chancellor's commitment to the HRA was clear (see Box 7.2). Though Lord Falconer did not rule out the possibility of issuing further guidance regarding the way in which the various articles of the European Convention on Human Rights (ECHR) should be applied, there would be no repeal of the HRA or withdrawal from the Convention. What the Lord Chancellor had been offering was further training and non-statutory guidance on how precisely the HRA should be applied by the police and other law enforcement agencies.

Box 7.2	Falconer defends the HRA

The Lord Chancellor insisted yesterday that Britain will not leave the European Convention on Human Rights or repeal the Human Rights Act. Lord Falconer warned that criticism of the judges for their human rights rulings risked undermining judicial independence.

Source: Clare Dyer, 'Lord Chancellor defends Britain's commitment to human rights', *Guardian*, 17 May 2006.

By 2009, however, Labour's approach had changed somewhat in both tone and scope. There was to be a new British Bill of Rights and Responsibilities that would build on those essential guarantees provided in the HRA. The Green Paper published in March 2009 provoked intense discussion and widespread criticism, with the then Lord Chancellor, Jack Straw, ultimately forced to concede that no progress would be made in advance of the next general election, amid rumours of a Cabinet revolt over the issue. The content of the Green Paper was, in fact, remarkably unremarkable, even when read through the blue-tinted spectacles of the *Daily Mail* (see Box 7.3).

The Conservatives' approach

From almost the beginning of his time as party leader, David Cameron offered a more root-and-branch approach to tackling what he saw as the defects of the HRA, than that proposed by the incumbent Labour government. Though initially suggesting that a Conservative government would 'reform, replace or scrap' the Act, the Conservative Party's position became far clearer in

Box 7.3   The *Daily Mail* on Labour's Green Paper

OBEY THE LAW... AND PAY YOUR TAXES	
The Human Rights Act gives Britons the following rights:	Yesterday's Green Paper suggests adding the following rights:
■ to life ■ not to be tortured, enslaved or made to carry out forced labour ■ to liberty and security ■ to a fair trial ■ to privacy and family life ■ to freedom of thought, conscience, religion and expression ■ to freedom of assembly and association ■ to marry ■ to the protection of property ■ to education ■ to free elections	■ to welfare ■ to free healthcare ■ to free education ■ to equality ■ to children's wellbeing ■ to a sustainable environment
	In return, citizens would be obliged to:
	■ treat public sector staff with respect ■ live in a 'green' way ■ vote and perform jury service ■ report crimes to the police ■ pay taxes and obey the law

Source: Benedict Brogan, 'Humiliation as Jack Straw ditches Labour's unworkable Bill of Rights pledge', *Daily Mail* (online), 23 March 2009.

2006 (see Boxes 7.4 and 7.5). Labour's initial preference for fine-tuning and additional guidance for those engaged in the administration of justice implied a failure to apply the HRA effectively as opposed to more fundamental flaws in the legislation. The Conservatives now appear committed to replacing, as opposed to amending or developing, the existing HRA.

Box 7.4   Cameron and the HRA

We need a new approach:
- The Human Rights Act has made it harder to protect our security.
- It is hampering our fight against crime and terrorism.
- It has done little to protect out liberties.
- It has helped create rights without responsibilities.

Source: David Cameron, 'Balancing freedom and security — a modern British Bill of Rights', 26 June 2006.

Cameron's preference is for a 'modern British Bill of Rights' (see Box 7.5) that would offer greater clarity than that present in the current HRA. In favouring clear but limited guarantees over the 'vague general principles' Cameron felt were enshrined in the HRA, such a Bill of Rights would, it was argued, leave senior judges significantly less room for interpretation.

Are such proposals warranted?

Though supporters of the HRA argue that it simply brings into British law those freedoms and rights previously available to British citizens under the ECHR, the application of these guarantees since the HRA came into force in October 2000 has given cause for concern. A particular worry has been the extent to which the Act has been used by those who engender little public sympathy, specifically criminals and foreign nationals facing deportation (see Box 7.6).

> ## Box 7.6   Does the HRA make any difference?
>
> Most lawyers reckon that the [Human Rights] Act, which was passed on Mr Blair's watch, simply codifies principles, such as the right to a fair trial...that were already in English law. Its opponents disagree. As well as protecting the rights of hijackers, they say, the Human Rights Act has given unreserved rights to murderers and made it impossible to deport criminals to countries where they might be in danger. The *Sun* newspaper, which has a Blair-like ear for public opinion, has set up a hotline for readers to call if they want to undo the Act, and has printed mugshots of troublesome judges.
>
> Source: 'The judges v. the government — wigging out', *The Economist*, 20 May 2006.

Such concerns, while entirely understandable, strike to the very heart of what a measure such as the HRA is supposed to do in terms of making fundamental rights available universally. The whole point of codifying such rights in this way is to protect those who might be denied their liberty under a less clearly laid out system (see Box 7.7).

While it is true that the HRA has seen the senior judiciary coming into conflict with government ministers on a more regular basis than was previously the case in the UK, this is an inevitable part of creating a 'rights culture' in the UK — and, moreover, a consequence that should surely not have been

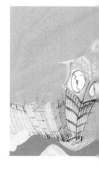

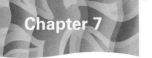

Box 7.7   In defence of the HRA

The Labour government has every reason to be proud of the Human Rights Act. In 1997 the then Home Secretary Jack Straw described the Act's passage through Parliament as 'an historic day'. Yet, last December, Straw, now Justice Secretary, declared that he was 'frustrated' by the way that the courts had interpreted the Act, encouraging a perception that it is 'a villain's charter'. Scrapping the HRA would send a terrible signal around the world that rights can be set aside when they prove too inconvenient or unpopular.

Source: Ben Ward, 'This insidious assault on the Human rights Act', *Independent*, 9 February 2009.

entirely unforeseen. Though the attacks of 9/11 and 7/7 and the anti-terror legislation that came after each attack have raised serious questions regarding the proper relationship between the judiciary and politicians, it is a function of an independent judiciary to protect citizens from a government that seeks to erode their rights. This observation is particularly true in respect of the judicial criticism of the use of the indefinite detention without trial of terrorist suspects under the Anti-terrorism, Crime and Security Act (2001), and the imposition of control orders, under the Prevention of Terrorism Act (2005). Both measures struck at the heart of the presumption of innocence, the right to a free and fair trial, and the freedom from arbitrary arrest. The belief of successive Labour home secretaries that the judges 'don't get it' (as John Reid put it) or are 'confused on rights' (as Charles Clarke claimed), reflects their genuine concern and frustration. It also betrays a failure to see the bigger picture.

Factfile   Derogation

A process by which a country is exempted, perhaps temporarily, from observing a law or regulation it had previously agreed to abide by.

Ultimately, of course, the government is not required to give way under pressure from judges. Declarations of incompatibility issued under the HRA only invite Parliament (more specifically, the government) to reconsider its position — a freedom to differ that has been apparent over control orders (see Box 7.8). We should also remember that the government can apply to derogate some of the guarantees enshrined in the ECHR in times of national emergency.

Box 7.8   Ignoring the courts?

The Home Office said that 'the ruling will not limit the operation of the Act. We will not be evoking either [this] control order, or any of the other control orders... in force'.

Source: 'Terror law an affront to justice — judge', *Guardian*, 29 June 2006.

What problems might such proposals present?

The problem of what to include in a new British Bill of Rights
The US Bill of Rights — referring collectively to the first ten amendments to the US constitution — is often championed as a model of how essential rights can be enshrined in a single document. In reality, however, it is a rather uneven document which combines guarantees of basic freedoms such as those outlined in the First and Fifth Amendments with other measures that today appear at best out of date (e.g. the Third Amendment) and at worst unhelpful (e.g. the Second Amendment). Moreover, this Bill of Rights did not include a prohibition of slavery (added with the 13th Amendment) or a guarantee of equal protection under the law (later included in the 14th Amendment). The question of precisely what should be included in a new British Bill of Rights is one that is likely to prove difficult to answer. The beauty of the UK's Human Rights Act was that it effectively sidestepped the need for a discussion over the fundamentals of what should be included by simply bringing a pre-existing list of rights and liberties — the ECHR — into British law.

The problem of how to engage the broader public in meaningful consultation
This problem of precisely what to include in a British Bill of Rights has prompted both major parties to suggest a kind of 'national conversation' or, as Labour put it, 'a dialogue with the British public'. Quite what this would mean in practice is unclear in a nation of over 60 million souls. A formal consultation along the lines that normally accompanies a Green Paper would surely fall way short of the kind of popular engagement and participation both parties are looking to encourage, as such processes are dominated by organised interests. The alternative, some kind of democratically appointed constitutional convention of the type employed at Philadelphia in 1787, appears equally improbable. Quite how David Cameron will achieve the 'national consensus' on the issue he says will be necessary in order to proceed is unclear. Perhaps this is another area in which the populist rhetoric of the two main UK parties will struggle to take on a concrete form.

The problem of what to do about the European Convention on Human Rights
The repeal of the HRA would not, of course, deny UK citizens access to the rights it guarantees because these same rights are enshrined in the ECHR, on which the HRA was based and to which the UK has been a signatory since the 1950s (see Box 7.9). Removing the HRA would, in effect, simply turn the clock back to a time when UK citizens would have to take their grievances to the European Court of Human Rights in Strasbourg. Though there is nothing to prevent the UK from withdrawing from the Convention entirely, such a course of action would be problematic: though remaining a party to the ECHR

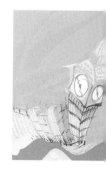

is not a legal requirement of EU membership, all of the 27 EU member states in 2009 were signatories.

Box 7.9   A 'pick-and-mix' approach to the ECHR

Parliament can repeal the entire Human Rights Act, but the UK would still be bound by the European Convention on Human Rights. There has been uninformed talk about 'renegotiating' part of the Convention, as if it were some list which asks countries to tick the rights they are prepared to grant and put crosses next to those they do not like. To have a sort of custom-built package of rights just for the Brits is absurd.

Source: Marcel Berlins, 'Stop blaming the Human Rights Act', *Guardian*, 15 May 2006.

Is it possible to have a meaningful Bill of Rights in the absence of a properly codified and entrenched constitution?

As a regular piece of statute law, the HRA can be amended or repealed like any other. In addition, we have already noted that under Article 15 of the ECHR national governments are permitted to derogate some of the Convention's articles in certain circumstances. For example, Part 4 of the UK's Anti-terrorism, Crime and Security Act (2001), authorising indefinite detention of foreign terrorist suspects, was only passed after the government opted to derogate Article 5 of the ECHR on the grounds that there was a 'public emergency threatening the life of the nation' (a form of words set out under Article 15).

Though the creation of a new British Bill of Rights would remove the second problem, as it would be entirely separate from the ECHR, the first problem would remain as a result of the doctrine of parliamentary sovereignty. In the absence of a 'higher law' — a properly codified and entrenched constitution — Parliament would always be free to alter or suspend the freedoms and liberties set out in such a Bill of Rights. Back in 2006, David Cameron suggested that a form of partial entrenchment might be achieved by adding the new Bill of Rights to the list of measures that the Commons cannot force through the Lords under the authority of the Parliament Act. Though such an obstacle, he argued, would not absolutely prevent a government from tinkering, it would present an additional level of protection for the measure.

Some argue that concerns over a lack of entrenchment are largely unfounded, as the Commons will always be reluctant to encroach upon those rights identified for fear of a public backlash. Thus, the new Bill of Rights might in time become so embedded in the public consciousness that no government would dare to tamper with it, even though Parliament would ultimately retain the authority to do so. In a sense, this process can be seen with the government ultimately backing down over indefinite detention and also in the failure of efforts to amend the Freedom of Information Act (2000) in such a way as to block access to details of MPs' expenses.

Conclusions: 'if it ain't broke...'

Codified and universal guarantees of rights and freedoms inevitably give rise to public controversy, as well as empowering the judiciary. One only needs to look to the example of the 'free speech' clause of the First Amendment to the US Constitution — a guarantee that the US Supreme Court has interpreted to protect everything from pure speech, through flag desecration, to semi-nude erotic dancing. Just as those who drafted the First Amendment might look back and wonder where it all went wrong, so might the Labour architects of the HRA engage in public soul-searching. The reality is, however, that the US Bill of Rights has become historically significant over the last 200 years, and the passage of the HRA might yet come to be seen as the 'historic' moment Jack Straw hailed back in 1997. Sadly, the prevailing public mood and the lack of entrenchment afforded to the HRA means that, unlike the US Bill of Rights, it will probably not survive long enough to be seen in this positive light.

Summary

- Both of the two main UK parties approached the 2010 general election with a commitment to respond to widespread public concern over the application of the Human Rights Act (HRA).
- Labour favoured developing it into a British Bill of Rights and Responsibilities, whereas the Conservatives looked to remove the HRA and put a British Bill of Rights in its place.
- Such proposals carry with them a number of problems, specifically what to include in this new Bill of Rights and how to afford it a degree of entrenchment (i.e. protection) in the absence of a codified and entrenched constitution.
- Scrapping the HRA will not remove the UK's obligations under the European Convention on Human Rights, and withdrawing from that Convention is not a realistic course of action.
- A single decade is too short a period over which to judge the worth of such a potentially historic measure — but time is clearly running out for the HRA.

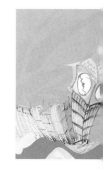

Chapter 8

Devolution at ten in Scotland and Wales: where to from here?

Context

The tenth anniversary of devolution in Scotland and Wales was marked by the publication of two reports. The first, the Calman Commission's Report on Scottish Devolution, addressed the performance of devolved institutions in Scotland since they opened for business back in 1999 and made recommendations on the future of governance north of the border. The second, the first report of the Independent Commission on Funding and Finance for Wales, took on the narrower remit of examining the way in which the Barnett Formula affects governance in the principality.

This chapter evaluates the performance of devolved government in Scotland and Wales in the light of these reports. In so doing it will address questions such as:
- What did the Calman Commission observe and what changes did it recommend?
- What is the Barnett Formula and why does it provoke such controversy?
- In what ways might devolution in Scotland and Wales be regarded as a success?
- What problems remain?
- Where to from here for devolution in Scotland and Wales?

What did the Calman Commission observe and what changes did it recommend?

The final report of the Calman Commission, a body established jointly by the UK government and the Scottish Parliament, delivered a very positive assessment of the first 10 years of devolution north of the border (see Box 8.1). Though problems clearly still remain — as we will see later in this chapter — the Commission largely accepted that which had been established by any number of opinion polls in recent years; namely, that most Scots approve of

| Box 8.1 | The Calman Commission's verdict |

Devolution has been a real success. The last 10 years have shown that not only is it possible to have a Scottish Parliament inside the UK, but that it works well in practice.... The Scottish Parliament has embedded itself in both the constitution of the United Kingdom and the consciousness of the Scottish people. It is here to stay.

Source: *Serving Scotland Better: Scotland and the United Kingdom in the 21st Century*, June 2009.

the work undertaken by the devolved institutions and that devolution is here to stay — having become 'embedded' in the national 'consciousness'.

Such a positive verdict on the process thus far inevitably meant that the Commission focused more on the ways in which devolution might be extended, than on any remedial action.

The report made a number of significant recommendations. Recommendation 3.1 would see the replacement of the Scottish Variable Rate of income tax with a new Scottish rate of income tax. Though this falls some way short of the financial independence sought by the Scottish Nationalists as a staging-post to full independence, it is clearly a small step along the same path. The devolution of taxes such as Stamp Duty Land Tax, Landfill Tax and Air Passenger Duty under recommendation 3.2, accompanied by a reduction in the block grant paid to Scotland by the UK government, should be seen in a similar light. Recommendation 4.15 (see Box 8.2) even hints at an extension of the Scottish Parliament's legislative powers.

Box 8.2 **Recommendation 4.15**

A new legislative procedure should be established to allow the Scottish Parliament to seek the consent of the UK Parliament to legislate in reserved areas where there is interaction with the exercise of devolved powers.

Source: *Serving Scotland Better: Scotland and the United Kingdom in the 21st Century*, June 2009.

What is the Barnett Formula and why does it provoke such controversy?

Introduced in 1978 and named after the then chief secretary to the Treasury, Joel Barnett, the Barnett Formula is part of the mechanism under which government spending for Scotland, Wales and Northern Ireland is determined. In simple terms, the formula works on the basis that any change in public expenditure in one part of the UK will result in a similar change in other areas, in proportion to their population.

The impact of the formula is hotly disputed. Whereas critics in Scotland and Wales lament the way in which it serves to bring about a closing of the gap between per-capita expenditure in England and Scotland (a process referred to as 'the Barnett Squeeze'), changes in population can at times result in the gap widening (as seen in Table 8.1).

English critics of the way in which funds are distributed between the nations that comprise the UK focus on two perceived faults in the system. First, that English taxpayers still receive more than £2,000 per capita less in government spending than those in Northern Ireland, c. £1,500 per capita less than those in Scotland, and c. £1,000 less than those in Wales (see also Table 8.1). Second, that the Barnett Formula gives the Scots in particular the benefit of government spending that they have chosen not to fund through taxation or other levies.

Table 8.1 *Government funding per capita, 2001–09 (UK = 100)*

Year	England	Wales	Scotland	N. Ireland
2001–02	96	112	119	132
2002–03	96	113	118	133
2003–04	97	113	117	126
2004–05	97	111	114	126
2005–06	97	111	117	124
2006–07	97	112	118	123
2007–08	97	111	118	125
2008–09	97	111	116	122

Source: House of Lords Select Committee on the Barnett Formula.

Neither phenomenon is particularly novel. As we saw in our 2007 survey, the first cause of concern was at the forefront of John Major's mind when tackling the issue of Scottish funding. As he recorded in his autobiography, 'Scotland already received 25 per cent more per head than England…I feared…that by exposing the reality of the favourable spending treatment given to Scotland, devolution would stir up latent English nationalist resentment leading to a backlash.' Our 2007 survey also highlighted an example of the second fault identified: that Scottish universities would get the benefit of top-up fees even though they had not been introduced in Scotland — because the benefit to English institutions was regarded as 'additional spending' under the Barnett Formula.

Perceptions of government funding in Scotland and Wales

These 'English criticisms' are covered in earlier surveys so there is no need for us to revisit them again here in great detail. What is of more relevance, however, is the Scottish and Welsh perspectives on funding inequality.

An ICM poll for BBC Scotland taken in June 2009 showed that many Scots feel that they lose out as a result of the funding arrangements in place (see Box 8.3). Though this perception is hardly surprising (it would surely be more shocking for people to agree that they should get less) it hints at one of the problems in the application of the Barnett Formula. That is, that the formula only works on changes in expenditure — it does not address expenditure as a whole or the relative needs of different areas. Thus while English taxpayers may appear to be subsidising the Scots and the Welsh to the tune of over £1,000 per capita, per annum, those on the receiving end may still feel that they are losing out, either because the rate of increased spending they are receiving under the formula is less than that enjoyed in England or because the funding formula does not recognise the particular funding needs of their community. The second problem is illustrated by the fact that government spending in different English regions — not governed by the Barnett Formula — varies wildly. London, for example, receives a per-capita spend close to that enjoyed by Scotland at 114% of the UK figure (see Table 8.1 for comparison). The North East receives around 111%, broadly in line with Wales, while the more affluent South East region — though contributing massively in terms of tax receipts — only receives around 85% of the UK-wide figure.

| Box 8.3 | Scottish perceptions of government spending |

Q Would you say that compared with other parts of the United Kingdom, Scotland gets pretty much its fair share of government spending, more than its fair share, or less than its fair share of government spending?

	Total	Men	Women
Pretty much its fair share	37	36	38
More than its fair share	12	15	9
Less than its fair share	43	44	43
Don't know	8	6	10

Source: ICM poll for BBC Scotland, June 2009.

The Barnett Formula's failure to fund the various nations that make up the UK on the basis of need — as is the norm for the English regions — is a major cause of concern for those feeling the full effect of the Barnett Squeeze in Scotland and Wales. In its first report, published in July 2009, the Independent Commission on Funding and Finance for Wales (see Box 8.4) estimated that the Barnet Formula would result in the principality being underfunded by *c.* £300 million in 2011–12, rising to between £5 billion and £9 billion by 2020–21, depending on the rate at which government spending rose. The commission's recommendation, that Wales should be funded at 114% of the English figure until a new system could be adopted, would mark a significant increase in the funding Wales received in 2008–09. That said, it would only provide the sort of funding that Wales would receive if it were funded in the same manner as English regions as opposed to under the Barnett Formula.

| Box 8.4 | Government funding in Wales |

The Barnett Formula...has no stated purpose other than getting a distribution done. In this it unquestionably succeeds. The purpose that can be inferred from its operation is to achieve the distribution with a minimum of public political conflict.

[However] our analysis has shown that Wales currently receives less than it would were it to be funded by the UK government using the formulae it applies to England.

Source: *Funding Devolved Government in Wales: Barnett and Beyond*, the First Report of the ICFFW, July 2009.

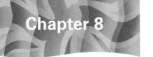

In what ways might devolution in Scotland and Wales be regarded as a success?

The Scottish experience

Support for devolution north of the border has remained relatively high (see Box 8.5). This is due, in no small part, to the populist policies adopted by the various Scottish administrations in office since 1999: it is difficult to imagine significant proportions of the population arguing against the provision of free nursing care for the elderly, the reduction and eventual abolition of prescription charges, the cancelling of toll charges across the Skye Toll Bridge or the reintroduction of beavers.

Box 8.5   Scottish perceptions of devolution

Q   Do you think that devolution has been a good thing for Scotland, a bad thing, or has it made no difference one way or the other?

	Total	Men	Women
Good thing	41	47	36
Bad thing	9	8	10
No difference	46	43	49
Don't know	3	2	5

Q   Do you think that as a result of having the Scottish Parliament, the health service in Scotland has got better, got worse, or has it not made much difference either way?

	Total	Men	Women
Got better	33	36	30
Got worse	9	8	10
No difference	52	50	54
Don't know	7	7	6

Q   Do you think that as a result of having the Scottish Parliament, standards in Scotland's schools have got better, got worse, or has it not made much difference either way?

	Total	Men	Women
Got better	29	31	28
Got worse	12	10	13
No difference	41	43	39
Don't know	18	17	20

Source: ICM poll for BBC Scotland, June 2009.

Although the SNP minority administration in power since 2007 has failed to achieve all that it set out to do — struggling even to secure the passage of its budget on occasion — there is no doubt that Scots have seen clear benefits from having so many aspects of everyday life controlled by devolved institutions; not least in the areas of healthcare and education (see Box 8.5).

The success of devolution can also be seen in the relatively low levels of support for full independence among Scots. The ICM poll for BBC Scotland taken in June 2009 (see Box 8.6) showed that while 38% would vote in favour of independence in the event of a referendum — slightly more than the one in four who favoured independence back in 2007 — the majority still favour Scotland remaining within the Union.

Box 8.6 Demand for independence

Q Are you in favour or against the idea of holding a referendum next year on whether Scotland should become independent?

	Total	Men	Women
In favour	58	62	55
Against	37	34	39
Don't know	5	3	6

Q In a referendum on independence for Scotland, how would you vote?

	Total	Men	Women
In favour	38	44	33
Against	54	50	58
Don't know	7	6	8
Refused	1	1	2

Source: ICM poll for BBC Scotland, June 2009.

The Welsh experience

Measuring the success of devolution in Wales is made more difficult first by the fact that the margin of victory for the 'yes' camp was so small at the time of the 1997 referendum and second by the fact that the secondary legislative powers afforded to the Welsh Assembly are so much more modest than those granted to the Scottish Parliament. Indeed, while the Calman Commission was able to conclude that devolution in Scotland had become embedded in the consciousness of the Scottish nation, an ICM poll for BBC Cymru Wales in February 2009 showed that fewer than 50% of Welsh adults even knew that the Welsh Assembly and Executive were controlled by Labour and Plaid Cymru's One Wales coalition (see Box 8.7), while 19% favoured abolishing the Assembly altogether — thereby bringing devolution in Wales to an abrupt end.

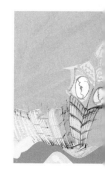

| Box 8.7 | Awareness of devolved arrangements in Wales |

Q Who do you think forms the current Welsh Assembly government?

	Total	Men	Women
Labour and Plaid Cymru	48	53	43
Labour	21	18	24
Plaid Cymru	6	6	6
Labour and the Liberal Democrats	5	6	5
Plaid Cymru and the Liberal Democrats	3	4	2
The Liberal Democrats	2	3	2
The Conservatives	2	1	2
Other	2	1	3
Don't know	11	9	13

Source: ICM poll for BBC Cymru Wales, February 2009.

Placing these negative findings to one side, however, there is clearly broad approval both for the work the Welsh Assembly and Executive have done since 1999 and — to a lesser degree — for the powers of devolved institutions in Wales to be brought into line with their Scottish counterparts (see Box 8.8). Most encouragement came from the finding that 40% of those questioned thought that the Assembly already had the most influence over Wales (with 29% favouring the Westminster Parliament), and 61% thought that the Assembly should have the most influence (21% for Westminster).

It would appear, therefore, that support for devolution in Wales is a good deal stronger now than it was a decade ago and this can only reflect favourably on the work that the Welsh Assembly and Executive have done, not least in promoting Welsh culture, abolishing prescription charges and tackling the thorny issue of university tuition fees.

What problems remain?

Original problems

The main problems present at the time that New Labour launched its devolution programme remain largely untouched. The decision to reduce the number of Scottish constituencies returning MPs to Westminster from 72 to 59 ahead of the 2005 general election was said to offer some partial solution to the West Lothian question (see factfile), but the reality is that it has done nothing of the kind.

Scotland is still over-represented at Westminster in relation to its population and the 59 MPs who can sit and vote in the capital are still often voting on measures that have little or no relevance to their constituents; whose everyday

Box 8.8 — The Welsh view on extending devolution

Q If there were to be a referendum on turning the National Assembly of Wales into a full law-making Welsh Parliament, how would you vote?

	Total	Men	Women
Yes	52	50	53
No	39	43	35
Don't know	9	6	11
Refused	0	0	1

Q Which one of these statements comes closest to your view?

	Total	Men	Women
Wales should become independent, separate from the UK and the EU	5	4	5
Wales should become independent, separate from the UK but part of the EU	8	8	7
Wales should remain part of the UK with its own elected parliament which has law-making and taxation powers	34	31	36
Wales should remain part of the UK, with its own elected parliament which has law-making *but no* taxation powers	10	10	10
Wales should remain part of the UK with its own elected assembly which has limited law-making powers only (as it has now)	21	20	22
Wales should remain part of the UK and the assembly should be abolished	19	22	16
None of these	0	0	0
Don't know	4	4	4

Source: ICM poll for BBC Cymru Wales, February 2009.

Factfile — The West Lothian question

- This refers to the fact that in many areas of policy, MPs representing Scottish constituencies at Westminster still have a say over policies that do not directly affect their own constituents, while having no say over most of the things that do, such powers having been devolved to the Scottish Parliament.
- First raised by the then Labour MP for West Lothian, Tam Dalyell, in the 1970s. Subsequently dubbed the West Lothian question by fellow MP Enoch Powell.
- Particularly apparent in the areas of education and healthcare.

Source: adapted from *A–Z Politics Handbook*, Philip Allan Updates, 2010.

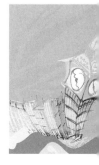

lives are governed largely from Holyrood. Though devolution in Wales presents less of a problem in this respect — as the Westminster Parliament retains legislative power in the principality — any decision to bring Welsh institutions into line with the Scottish Parliament would create exactly the same problem, a 'Blaenau Gwent question', perhaps.

New problems

The various facets of the West Lothian question have been discussed, if not resolved, for over 30 years, but other problems have become apparent over the first decade that devolution has been in operation:

First, the failure of devolution in England — more specifically the failure to establish directly elected English regional assemblies — has resulted in a form of asymmetrical devolution that appears untenable in the short to medium term, yet alone the long term.

Second, there has been a marked divergence in the application of certain highly visible public policies across the various home nations. This is most notable in the case of prescription charges — those resident in England are likely to be the only UK citizens who will have to pay for prescription medication by 2011.

These new problems have resulted in growing resentment in England and — paradoxically — an increase for the cause of Scottish independence among the English just as the Scots themselves are becoming less enamoured with the concept.

Conclusions: where to from here for devolution in Scotland and Wales?

Some people have characterised the situation created by devolution in Scotland and Wales as a form of quasi-federalism, a mid-way point between the unitary form of government traditionally practised in the UK and the style of federalism under which countries such as the USA and Germany operate. However, Vernon Bogdanor, writing in *Politics Review,* Vol. 19, No. 3, saw things rather differently: whereas the various states under a federal system remain part of the larger nation, he argued, the UK is in fact emerging as a 'nation of nations' — each with 'its own identity and institutions'.

Precisely where the process that has led to the emergence of this 'nation of nations' will ultimately lead is, as yet, unclear. The ICM polls of 2009 showed that while 58% of Scots would like a referendum on full independence, only 38% would vote in favour if given the opportunity to do so. In Wales the picture is starker still, with just 13% favouring independence from the UK and only 34% wanting to bring Wales into line with Scotland by turning the Welsh Assembly into a parliament with primary legislative and tax-varying powers.

Thus, far from being the thin end of a wedge designed to divide the constituent parts of the UK, devolution has in fact underpinned support for the Union in both Scotland and Wales. In Wales, the limited support for independence is perhaps rooted in historical and socioeconomic realities: the fact that Wales is simply not viable as a wholly independent entity. In Scotland, the reality is more subtle, for the extensive primary legislative powers afforded to the Scottish Parliament might already be said to have created an independence of sorts (see Box 8.9).

Box 8.9   The reality in Scotland?

The fact that support for full independence has fallen to only one in four of Scots since the SNP came to power rather misses the point. As Channel 4's Stuart Cosgrove commented in the *Guardian* (15 November 2007), 'a lot of [the debate over independence] feels so arcane.... The truth of the matter is, apart from some key institutions maybe it's already happened. That's the thing: Scotland already is independent, isn't it?'

Source: 'What's New', *Politics Review*, Vol. 17, No. 4.

Summary

- Devolution in Scotland and Wales is largely seen as a New Labour success story, with high levels of popular support for the work of devolved institutions in both countries.
- The way in which government spending is divided between the various home nations — most notably the operation of the Barnett Formula — remains a bone of contention on all sides.
- Tam Dalyell's fears regarding devolution — as encapsulated in the West Lothian question — have largely been borne out by events since the establishment of devolved government in Scotland.
- Extending devolution in Wales would run the risk of duplicating such problems — in effect, creating a 'Blaenau Gwent question'.
- While some argue that devolution has created a kind of quasi-federalism, Vernon Bogdanor argues that we are in fact seeing the emergence of a new 'nation of nations'.
- There appears to be little appetite for full independence in either Scotland or Wales.

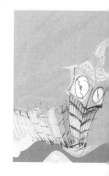